"*The Probiotic Solution* is an excellent guide for readers who want to expand their knowledge of probiotics and the new findings emerging from current research."
—**Dallas Clouatre, Ph.D.**, author of *The Prostate Miracle* and *Anti-Fat Nutrients*

"As powerful tools in the prevention and treatment of certain conditions, probiotics will play an increasingly important role in human health. *The Probiotic Solution* highlights one of the most beneficial, science-based nutraceuticals around in a concise, consumer-friendly way. Here's to the "good guys"!"
—**Rebecca Madley**, Editor, *Nutraceuticals World*

"*The Probiotic Solution* offers new and exciting perspectives on probiotics and their potential for improving health. Dr. Brudnak shows an insight into the root causes of many maladies that have largely been ignored by the medical community. *The Probiotic Solution* explores the symbiotic relationship these friendly bacteria provide in disease prevention and health maintenance."
—**James Roza C.N.**, NOW Foods

"I have found that when there is dysbiosis (overgrowth of yeast, bacteria and/or viruses) in the intestinal tract that my patients have greater problems with intestinal permeability (leaky gut), food allergies, chemical sensitivities, immune suppression and inflammatory reactions. An important key to solving these problems has been the use of broad-spectrum probiotics that enhance digestion, strengthen intestinal immune function, and support internal healing."
— **Dr. Roy Kerry**, Advanced Integrative Medicine Center

THE PROBIOTIC SOLUTION

Nature's Best-Kept Secret for Radiant Health

Dr. Mark A. Brudnak

Published in the United States by:
Dragon Door Publications, Inc
P.O. Box 4381, St. Paul, MN 55104
Tel: (651) 487-2180
Fax: (651) 487-3954
Credit card orders: 1-800-899-5111
Email: dragondoor@aol.com
Website: www.dragondoor.com

Book design, Illustrations and cover by Derek Brigham
Website http//www.dbrigham.com
Tel/Fax: (612) 827-3431
Email: dbrigham@visi.com

Manufactured in the United States
First Edition: May 2003

Many of the designations used by manufacturers and sellers to distinguish their products are claimed as trademarks. Where those designations appear in this book and the publisher was aware of a trademark claim, the designations have been printed in caps or initial caps.

Genomeceuticals is a trademark belonging to MAK Wood, Inc. Grafton, WI.

The statements contained in this book have not been evaluated by the Food and Drug Administration. The products are not intended to diagnose, treat, cure, or prevent any disease. This information is provided for your guidance only and is not intended as medical information, recommendations, or suggestions. Please consult a medical doctor for such information. We urge you to make all tests you deem appropriate. No warranties, expressed or implied, including warranties of merchantability or fitness for a particular purpose, are made regarding products described or information set forth, or that such products or information may be used with freedom from patent infringement.

DISCLAIMER
This book is for reference and informational purposes only and is in no way intended as medical counseling or medical advice. The information contained herein should not be used to treat, diagnose or prevent any disease or medical condition without the advice of a competent medical professional. The author and Dragon Door Publications shall have neither liability nor responsibility to any person or entity with respect to any loss, damage, or injury caused or alleged to be caused directly or indirectly by the information contained in this book.

Contents

What is cancer?...what happens when normal cells become cancerous... different cancers...what causes cancer?...risk factors and protective factors...the effects of tobacco...the role of diet in the development and prevention of cancer...UV radiation...alcohol...the dangers of ionizing radiation...chemicals and other substances...the dangers of Hormone Replacement Therapy and DES...genetics...how is cancer treated?... surgery...the perils of chemotherapy and radiotherapy...laser ablation... what is the Probiotic Solution?...DNA and mutations... unwrapping... probiotics as detoxifiers...as a physical barrier to bacteria...*bacteria adherence*...the internal politics of the intestines—the good, the bad and the ugly...the toxic battlefield...the species of probiotics in the normal GI tract...what's on the market...why taking probiotics is not a one-time fix...the ongoing war...the need for fresh troops.

CHAPTER 4: Why Probiotics May Spell Relief for Alzheimer's Disease   45

What is Alzheimer's disease?...what causes Alzheimer's disease...the amyloid cascade *hypothesis*...heavy metal toxicity...the *lock-and-key hypothesis of enzyme functionality*...when the Pac-Man enzyme can no longer eat the substrate...the killer advent of *cytoxic plaques*...how is Alzheimer's disease diagnosed and treated?...*neuropsychological* testing... imaging tests...medications...what is the probiotic solution?...the prophylactic and therapeutic benefits of phosphatidyl serine...reducing the accumulation of plaques...*mitochondrial dysfunction*...excess calcium and *signal transduction*...probiotics as a calcium stabilizer...the benefits of *isoflavones*.

CHAPTER 5: How Probiotics Can Help Counteract the Effects of Lactose Intolerance   55

What is lactose intolerance?...common symptoms...who is most likely to be lactose intolerant?...what causes lactose intolerance?...*Congenital-type lactose intolerance*...*adult-type lactose intolerance*...what is *lactose*? ...the role of *lactase*...diagnosis of lactose intolerance...the *lactose tolerance test*...the *hydrogen breath test*...cautions for infants...the *stool acidity* test...how is lactose intolerance treated?...good alternatives to straight dairy...hidden sources of lactose...what is the Probiotic Solution?...the function of the beta-gal enzyme...pathogenic feeding frenzies...fresh yogurt...survival rates...the importance of mixing probiotic strains...why resistant strains are not the best answer...optimal delivery systems...when to take probiotics...combining enzymes and probiotics.

CHAPTER 6: The Probiotics Potential for Diabetes and for Effective Weight Control   65

What is diabetes?...the two types of diabetes...type II—a major cause of heart disease, kidney disease, stroke, blindness, and early death...the intimate relationship between diabetes and weight control...what causes diabetes?...genetic and lifestyle factors...the role of insulin...the hormone *leptin* for appetite control...how is diabetes treated?...what is the Probiotic Solution?...the three basic strategies for treating diabetes ...reducing glucose absorption in the gastrointestinal (GI) tract...how to have your cake and eat it too...how glucose functions in the body...why probiotics prefer glucose...the relationship to glycogen...the dangers of yeast and *E. coli supplementation*...excess stored energy and weight gain... accelerating the metabolism of glucose with probiotics.

CHAPTER 10: Choosing The Best Probiotic Delivery Systems   109

Why it's all in the delivery...probiotics—ally in the war against disease and infection...changing the public perception about *good* bacteria...the traditional probiotic delivery system—fermented dairy products...plusses and minuses...what to look for...alternate probiotic delivery systems... how *prebiotics* add value to a delivery system....recommended prebiotics...the Brudnak Method of pulsing and rotating—the hows and whys...defining the "pulse"...the problem of *genetic drift*...clinical results with autism...recommended probiotic manufacturers and products...choosing the right probiotic for you—what to look for...where to buy probiotic products.

Foreword
by Dennis T. Gordon, Ph.D.

Professor, Institute of Food Technologist and Organizer of the 2002 IFT Basic Symposium "Dietary Fiber, Prebiotics, Probiotics and Their Role in Intestinal Health, " Department of Cereal Science, North Dakota State University

The idea of using probiotics has a long tradition, but modern science is just beginning to realize its benefits. It was Elie Metchnikoff's original view in 1907 that having a balanced microflora was best for a person's health. His theory can certainly be viewed as championing one of the most important recommendations for a good diet: that is, to eat a variety of foods, which should include fermented foods and now probiotics. In this book, *The Probiotic Solution*, Mark Brudnak helps us review and think of probiotics as nutraceuticals for the possible prevention and or treatment of other diseases.

Fermented foods provide food-safe organisms, and these foods and bacteria have provided some of the original concepts for *nutraceuticals* and *probiotics*, respectively. Today's probiotic organisms are rigorously selected and screened for numerous properties, which include vitality in the human intestine to complement intestinal functions and the microflora along the entire intestinal tract. Probiotics appear to "prime" the intestinal immune system and have been shown to have therapeutic application in the treatment of rotavirus-caused diarrhea and lactose intolerance.

In addition to having nutraceutical benefits, probiotics also serve as important biomarkers that help us better understand the total function of the intestine and importance of its microflora to other diseases. Probiotics may prove helpful in understanding and possibly preventing or treating intestinal infections—most notably, those caused by *Helicobacter pyloris*, chronic inflammatory bowel diseases, antibiotic-induced and traveler's diarrhea, pouchitis, atopic disease (asthma), and colon cancer.

Introduction

Many people believe that "Disease begins in the colon." While this is certainly true up to a point, it's *not* the complete truth. The complete truth is that good health results from producing a balance in the body. The converse of that is when the body is out of balance, disease sets in. So, it's the lack of balance in the body that causes disease and ultimately death.

Thus, there are as many causes of disease as there are causes of body imbalance. For instance, if there's too much of a cancer-causing agent (or carcinogen) in the body, then the imbalance results in cancer. If there's too much cholesterol in the body, then a disease such as coronary heart disease (CHD) results. If there are too many toxins in the body, then a condition such as diarrhea results. The list goes on and on, and for each disease state, if we look at it closely enough, we'll find an imbalance. It's a law of nature.

Reports from the medical community show that the major reason people visit the doctor is for some sort of gastrointestinal problem. Again, let's look closely at what's going on here. In our modern-day society, people are consuming tremendous amounts of processed foods. In fact, well over 90% of the average American's diet comes from processed foods! These foods are high in bad things, like bleached flour and artificial colors and flavors, and low in good things, like whole grains and vitamins and minerals. The result, of course, is an imbalance—and sooner or later, the disease that comes along with it. Clearly, we need to bring our bodies back in balance if we are going to protect our own lives along with those of our family members. We need to restore the balance that was there when our mothers first nursed us.

At birth, the human system is as perfect as it will ever be. Sure, things aren't completely formed yet, but as far as a life is considered, a newborn baby is the healthiest person on the planet! Slowly, as the environment we live in pollutes us, we begin to fall out of balance. Sometimes, this happens very quickly, and we get a condition such as diarrhea, but usually, the process is gradual and a more insidious disease strikes. It isn't until much later in life that we begin to notice the effects that really began in childhood.

And so, as we age, the effects of eating a poor diet and absorbing environmental toxins catch up with us. We start experiencing diseases such as arthritis, cancer, heart disease, and many more. Some diseases have even become alarmingly widespread among children. For example, there has been a dramatic increase in the level of type II diabetes in children as young as the early teens. Similarly, there has been an astronomical rise in the rate of autism over the past 10 years. This used to be a relatively rare disease, thought to affect 1 in 10,000 children. Now, it's believed that as many as 1 in 200 children may be autistic. This is amazing, and it's all due to the body being out of balance.

Make no mistake: This is a war! The potential causalities are not just you but also your family. Your children, husband or wife, parents and grandparents are all with you on the front line. A battle of epic proportions is raging inside each of them. What they are fighting is an unseen and unrelenting enemy that is viciously struggling to take control of their bodies—an enemy capable of unleashing the biological equivalent of an atomic bomb at any second and wiping out their lives! That enemy consists of deadly microbes, the so-called bad bacteria and viruses known as *germs*.

Without intervention, that enemy will ultimately win the battle and perhaps even the war. Your life, along with the lives of everyone you love, is in danger, but you don't have to surrender yet. There is a shimmer of white light on the battleground, so fear not! You can be the commander of the good forces. You can assay your troops and plan a counterattack that will rescue your family and lead to final victory. You have the ultimate weapon at your disposal! This book, *The Probiotic Solution*, will show you how to fight back.

Just as firefighters use fire to fight fire, you can use good bacteria to fight bad. Those good bacteria are known as probiotics and exist naturally in the human body. Probiotics are your friend and your weapon, your key to good health and your counter-balance against the bad forces in nature. Probiotics are the soldiers you have brought forth to fight the evil, disease-causing forces.

Probiotics consist of a number of different types of friendly microorganisms. They have assisted in maintaining the lives of humans (and other animals) since the beginning of time. However, they have been recognized as the true weapons in human health care only since the early 1900s. The pioneering work of Russian scientist Elie Metchnikoff (1845–1916) is largely responsible for this recognition. He noted that the Bulgarians in the Caspian Mountains lived extraordinarily long lives. In studying their culture, he found nothing out of the ordinary except for one thing: They drank a fermented milk product known as *kefir*. This observation gave rise to what is known as Metchnikoff's *longevity without aging theory*. The basic idea is that by ingesting a lot of good bacteria, or probiotics, the harmful effects of the bad bacteria can be negated or at least diminished.

We now know that kefir contains several types or strains of probiotics. Kefir is traditionally prepared by pouring fresh goat's milk into a large leather flask and then hanging it in the doorway. As people go in and out throughout the day, they give the flask a little push, which serves to stir up the mixture and aid in the fermentation process. Each day, they also take a little out, drink it, and then add more milk to fill the flask back up. This way, production is ongoing.

So, why doesn't everyone drink kefir? The problem is that it's proven difficult to make with any consistency. When scientists have tried to isolate the exact probiotics in the mixture, the results have varied from batch to batch. So, how would you know which batch to drink? Well, you wouldn't. Selecting the right one would result purely by chance. And while it's known that kefir contains various lactic acid bacteria and yeast, exactly which ones are responsible for any health benefits has remained elusive. (We will talk about the health benefits of various probiotics in more detail later.)

Most people don't realize that they are, in a sense, actually partaking in this ancient ritual when they consume products such as yogurt. Yogurt is very similar to kefir but usually contains other organisms. The main difference between kefir and yogurt has to do with the length of the fermentation process; specifically, that process is allowed to progress until the yogurt has formed.

Are yogurt and kefir the only sources of probiotics? Certainly not. Are they sufficient, in and of themselves, for promoting optimal health for you and your family? Absolutely not! Please remember that this is a war, and in all wars, numbers count. In the products commonly found in grocery stores, such as probiotic-supplemented milk and yogurt, the numbers of organisms are very low in comparison with the huge numbers of bad bacteria waging war in the bodies of you and your family members. While the products on the store shelves may start off with some live probiotics, chances are, by the time you eat those products, most of the live probiotics will be dead. This renders these products useless, because science has shown that equally large numbers of good bacteria are needed to fight off the bad.

Certainly, supplements are available that contain live probiotics. However, in recent tests of these supplements, they did not all pass. Many contained dead bacteria and even mislabeled products. Some even contained potentially deadly bacteria! How do you know which products to buy and which to pass over?

I devote an entire chapter (Chapter 10, Probiotic Delivery Systems) to explaining exactly what you need to know to arm yourself and your family when you go to select probiotic products at the store. Frankly, it's hard for us, as Westerners, to accept the idea of deliberately putting bacteria into our bodies when so much in our culture tells us of the need to kill bacteria and disinfect our lives. We must get over this and understand that there are such things as good and friendly bacteria and that consuming even billions of them at a time can be beneficial.

To be sure, other products in the market are capable of supplying the high numbers of live and functional probiotics you and your family need to win the war on disease. I discuss the ideas behind these products, including probiotic *type* (because which strains or types you can choose could mean the difference between wining or losing the war) and *viability* (or how alive the products are when you buy them). I also discuss the various diseases mentioned earlier (see Chapters 1–9) and the influence that probiotics have in their prevention and treatment. Finally, throughout the text, I provide sources you can turn to for more information (see the Resources and Bibliography, in particular).

Given the threat of global terrorism, and especially the potential for biological attacks, it is a relief to find out that there are good bacteria that can be used to fight bad bacteria. It has been demonstrated that even such horrendous bacteria as Bacillus anthracis, or anthrax, can be fought using probiotics. We can outnumber the invaders and force them out of the bodies of our children.

This book, *The Probiotic Solution*, is designed to be your war manual, your battle flag, your torch, and your shield. As such, it provides all the information you need not only to decide which probiotics are right for each member of your family but also to wisely deploy your troops, your friends, your probiotics. As you rally your troops and prepare to take back the health and well-being of your family, you will be armed with the knowledge of where the enemy is and what it is planning. This is a war you can win, and this book will show you how.

Recently, I spoke with Dr. Harry G. Preuss, professor of physiology, medicine, and pathology (tenured) at Georgetown University, who has an impressive list of qualifications in the area of nutrition. In particular, he has consulted for Novartis Pharmaceuticals (Summit, NJ), Alternet Health Technologies (Los Angeles, CA), and InterHealth Nutraceuticals

(Benicia, CA) about the nature of probiotics and their emerging recognition. Dr. Preuss has this to say about the gaining popularity of probiotics:

> The use of probiotics in nutritional supplements is in its infancy. With more books, such as *The Probiotic Solution*, to expand social awareness and acceptance, we are just at the beginning of what will be a hyperbolic curve for probiotic use.

I cannot overstate the importance of probiotics. To quote Dr. Dallas Clouatre, author of *The Prostate Miracle, Anti-Fat Nutrients*, and numerous other books:

> The gastrointestinal tract is the gateway for the entry of all substances into the body other than injected compounds or items brought in via the lungs. For this reason, probiotics and other supplements, which directly influence the health of the GI-tract can exert a powerful influence on the long- term status of the entire body. The uptake of nutrients is heavily influenced by the microbial population of the gut, and this influence extends to the absorption of minerals, such as calcium, that we do not normally realize is dependent upon the actions of probiotics.

My purpose in writing this book is best summed up by the famous Dr. Jonathan Collin, editor in chief of the *Townsend Letter for Doctors* and Patients, who said:

> The published peer-reviewed literature is in its infancy with regard to probiotics, and yet it is expansive. It seems to be growing at an almost exponential manner. It is now understood that probiotics may affect everything from various neurological symptoms to yeast infections. Scientists know this and the scientific community is at the stage where the popular literature, reaching the lay masses, has to get to get this information to them. As a society, we need to come to terms with the fact that what we look like physically on the inside is at least as important as what we look like on the outside. For instance, we know that by maintaining a proper probiotic population in the

gastrointestinal tract, we have a direct bearing on things such as Eczema. *The Probiotic Solution* takes information such as that and makes it accessible to the everyday person.

And finally, the trend toward probiotics is summed up nicely by Rebecca Madley, editor of *Nutraceuticals World*:

Probiotics are finally starting to hit the radar screen in terms of recognition in the marketplace. Over the next several years more scientific documentation of health benefits and better communication to the consumer will provide a more solid platform from which probiotic products can be expected to launch. As powerful tools in the prevention and treatment of certain conditions, in addition to providing regular maintenance of the gastrointestinal tract, probiotics will play an increasingly important role in human health.

CHAPTER 1

How Probiotics Can Help Solve the Cancer Problem

WHAT IS CANCER?

Cancer is a group of many related diseases that begin in the cells of the body, the basic unit of life. In short, it's the uncontrolled growth of cells that are derived from normal cells, and it can go on to kill off normal cells either at the original site or in other parts of the body. To understand cancer, it's helpful to know what happens when normal cells become cancerous.

The body is made up of many types of cells. Normally, cells grow and divide to produce more cells only when the body needs them. This orderly process helps keep the body healthy. Sometimes, however, cells keep dividing even when new cells are not needed. These extra cells form a mass of tissue called a *growth* or *tumor*.

A tumor can be *benign* or *malignant*. A benign tumor is not cancerous. It can often be removed and, in most cases, does not come back. Moreover, the cells from a benign tumor do not spread to other parts of the body. Most important, a benign tumor is rarely a threat to life. A *malignant* tumor is cancerous. The cells in this type of tumor are abnormal and divide without control or order. They can invade and damage nearby tissues and organs. Also, cancer cells can break away from a malignant tumor and enter the bloodstream or the lymphatic system. That's how cancer spreads from the original cancer site to form new tumors in other organs; this process is called *metastasis*. Leukemia and lymphoma are examples of cancers that arise in blood-forming cells.

Most cancers are named for the organ or type of cell in which they begin. For example, cancer that begins in the lung is *lung cancer*, and cancer that begins in cells in the skin, known as *melanocytes*, is called *melanoma*.

When cancer spreads, or metastasizes, from its original site, cancer cells are often found in nearby or regional lymph nodes (sometimes called *lymph glands*). If cancer cells have reached these nodes, it means that the cancer may have spread to other organs, such as the liver, bones, and brain. When cancer spreads from its original location to another part of the body, the new tumor has the same kind of abnormal cells and the same name as the primary tumor. For example, if lung cancer spreads to the brain, the cancer cells in the brain are actually lung cancer cells. The disease is called metastatic *lung cancer*, not *brain cancer*.

WHAT CAUSES CANCER?

The more we can learn about what *causes* cancer, the more likely we will find ways to prevent it. In the laboratory, scientists explore the possible causes of cancer and try to determine exactly what happens in cells when they become cancerous. Researchers also study patterns of cancer in the population to look for *risk factors*, or conditions that increase the chance that cancer might occur. In addition, researchers look for *protective factors*, or things that decrease the risk.

Although doctors can seldom explain why one person gets cancer and another does not, it's clear that cancer is not caused by an injury, such as a bump or bruise. And while being infected with certain viruses may increase the risks for some types of cancer, cancer is not contagious. No one can catch cancer from another person.

So, how does cancer develop? It develops over time as the result of a complex mix of factors related to lifestyle, heredity, and environment. Even so, a number of factors have been identified that increase a person's chance of developing cancer. (We will discuss these in detail in the next section.) For instance, many types of cancer are related to the use of tobacco, to what people eat and drink, to exposure to ultraviolet (UV) radiation from the sun, and to a lesser extent, exposure to cancer-causing agents (or *carcinogens*) in the environment and the workplace. Some people are more sensitive than others to these factors, yet most of the people who get cancer have *none* of the known risk factors. In addition, most people who *do* have risk factors do not get the disease.

Some cancer risk factors can be avoided. Others, such as inherited factors (for instance, having fair skin and being especially sensitive to UV radiation), are unavoidable, but it may be helpful to be aware of them. We can help protect ourselves by avoiding known risk factors whenever possible. We can also have regular checkups and talk with our doctors about whether cancer-screening tests could be of benefit.

CANCER RISK FACTORS

Tobacco. Smoking tobacco, using smokeless tobacco, and being regularly exposed to environmental tobacco smoke are responsible for one-third of all cancer deaths in the United States each year. This makes tobacco use the most preventable cause of death in the country.

Smoking accounts for more than 85 percent of all lung cancer deaths. For smokers, the risk of getting lung cancer increases with the amount of tobacco they smoke each day, the number of years they have smoked, the type of tobacco product they use, and how deeply they inhale. Overall, for someone who smokes one pack a day, the chance of getting lung cancer is about 10 times greater than that of a nonsmoker.

Cigarette smokers are also more likely than nonsmokers to develop several other types of cancer, including oral cancer and cancers of the larynx, esophagus, pancreas, bladder, kidney, and cervix. Smoking may also increase the likelihood of developing cancers of the stomach, liver, prostate, colon, and rectum. People who smoke cigars and pipes are at risk for cancers of the oral cavity about as much as people who smoke cigarettes. Cigar smokers also have an increased chance of developing cancers of the lung, larynx, esophagus, and pancreas. When a smoker quits, however, the risk of cancer soon begins to decrease and continues to decline gradually each year.

The use of smokeless tobacco products, such as chewing tobacco and snuff, may cause cancers of the mouth and throat. Precancerous conditions, or tissue changes that may lead to cancer, often begin to go away after a person stops using smokeless tobacco.

People who don't use tobacco products can also be at risk for smoking-related cancer. Studies suggest that exposure to environmental tobacco smoke, also called *secondhand smoke*, increases the risk of lung cancer for nonsmokers.

Someone who uses tobacco in any form and needs help quitting may want to talk with his or her doctor, dentist, or other health professional or join a smoking cessation group sponsored by a local hospital or voluntary organization. Information about finding such groups and programs is available from the Cancer Information Service (CIS). (For contact information, see the Resources section at the end of the book.) CIS information specialists can send printed materials and also give suggestions about quitting that are tailored to an individual caller's needs.

Diet. What is the role of diet in the development of cancer? Some evidence suggests a link between a high-fat diet and certain cancers, such as cancers of the colon, uterus, and prostate. Being seriously overweight may be linked to breast cancer among older women and to cancers of the prostate, pancreas, uterus, colon, and ovary in the general population. Other studies suggest that eating foods containing fiber and certain nutrients may help protect against some types of cancer.

We may be able to reduce our cancer risk by making healthy food choices. A well-balanced diet includes generous amounts of foods that are high in fiber, vitamins, and minerals and low in fat. This means eating a lot of fruits and vegetables and more whole-grain breads and cereals *every day*, along with fewer eggs and not as much high-fat meat, dairy products (such as whole milk, butter, and most cheeses), and oils (such as salad dressing, margarine, and cooking oil).

Most scientists think that making healthy food choices is more beneficial than taking vitamin and mineral supplements.

Ultraviolet (UV) Radiation. UV radiation from the sun causes premature aging of the skin and skin damage that can lead to skin cancer. Artificial sources of UV radiation, such as sunlamps and tanning booths, also can cause skin damage and probably increase the risk of getting skin cancer.

To help reduce the risk of skin cancer caused by UV radiation, it's best to reduce exposure to the midday sun (from 10 A.M. to 3 P.M.). Another simple rule is to avoid the sun at those times of day when your shadow is shorter than you are. Wearing a broad-brimmed hat, UV-absorbing sunglasses, long pants, and long sleeves offers additional protection.

Many doctors believe that, in addition to avoiding the sun and wearing protective clothing, wearing *sunscreen*—especially one that reflects, absorbs, and/or scatters the two main types of UV radiation (UVA and UVB)—may help prevent some forms of skin cancer. Sunscreens are rated in strength according to a *sun protection factor*, or SPF. The higher the SPF, the more sunburn protection that's provided. Sunscreens with SPFs of 12 through 29 are adequate for most people, when applied according to the directions. Typically, those directions recommend to apply sunscreen liberally and to reapply it after going in the water.

Regardless of the protective value of wearing sunscreen, it is not a substitute for avoiding the sun and wearing protective clothing.

Alcohol. Heavy drinkers have an increased risk of cancers of the mouth, throat, esophagus, larynx, and liver. People who smoke cigarettes and drink heavily are at especially high risk for these cancers. Some studies suggest that even moderate drinking may cause a slight increase in the risk of breast cancer.

Ionizing Radiation. Cells may be damaged by ionizing radiation from X-ray procedures, radioactive substances, rays that enter the earth's atmosphere from outer space, and other sources. In very high doses, ionizing radiation may cause cancer and other diseases. Studies of people who survived the dropping of atomic bombs in Japan during World War II show that ionizing radiation increases the risk of developing leukemia and cancers of the breast, thyroid, lung, stomach, and other organs.

Before 1950, X-rays were used to treat noncancerous conditions (such as an enlarged thymus, enlarged tonsils and adenoids, ringworm of the scalp, and acne) in children and young adults. Those who received radiation therapy to the head and neck have a higher-than-average risk of developing thyroid cancer. Anyone who has had such a treatment should report it to his or her doctor.

The radiation used as therapy to destroy cancerous cells can also damage normal cells. (See the section later in this chapter titled How Is Cancer Treated?) Before having such therapy, a patient should talk with his or her doctor about the effect of radiation treatment in terms of increasing the risk of getting a second cancer. This risk can depend on the patient's age at the time of treatment as well as on the part of the body to be treated.

The X-rays used to diagnose certain conditions (such as mammograms and dental X-rays) expose people to lower levels of radiation than those used for cancer therapy, and the benefits nearly always outweigh the risks. However, repeated exposure can be harmful, so it's a good idea to talk with your doctor about the need for each X-ray and to ask about the use of shields to protect other parts of the body.

Chemicals and Other Substances. Being exposed to certain chemicals, metals, and pesticides can also increase the risk of cancer. Asbestos, nickel, cadmium, uranium, radon, vinyl chloride, benzidene, and benzene are all examples of well-known carcinogens. Each may act alone or along with another carcinogen, such as cigarette smoke, to increase the risk of cancer. For example, inhaling asbestos fibers at work increases the risk of all lung diseases, including cancer, and for asbestos workers who smoke, that risk is especially high.

It's important to follow work and safety rules to avoid or minimize contact with dangerous materials. In most cases, employers are required by law to inform workers of the dangers from chemicals and other substances found in their work environment.

Hormone Replacement Therapy (HRT). Doctors may recommend HRT—using either *estrogen* alone or in combination with *progesterone*—to control the symptoms that may occur in women during menopause (such as hot flashes and vaginal dryness). Studies have shown that the use of estrogen alone increases the risk of cancer of the uterus. Therefore, most doctors prescribe HRT that includes progesterone along with low doses of estrogen. Progesterone counteracts estrogen's harmful effect on the uterus by preventing overgrowth of the lining of the uterus, which is associated with taking estrogen alone. (Estrogen alone may be prescribed for a woman who has had a *hysterectomy*, or surgery to remove the uterus, and is therefore not at risk for cancer of the uterus.) Other studies show an increased risk of breast cancer among women who have used estrogen for a long time, and some research suggests that the risk might be higher among those who have used estrogen and progesterone together. HRT has proven and presumable benefits for women who wish to preserve their postmenopausal health, including the prevention of bone loss and age-related dementia.

Researchers are still learning about the risks and benefits of taking HRT, and there is considerable debate about these issues. A woman considering HRT should do her best to be well informed and discuss these issues with her doctor.

Diethylstilbestrol (DES). DES is a synthetic form of estrogen that was used starting in the early 1940s and then discontinued in 1971.

Some women took DES during pregnancy to prevent certain complications, only to discover years later that doing so put their daughters at risk for certain cancers. DES-exposed daughters have an increased chance of developing abnormal cells (*dysplasia*) in the cervix and vagina and are also at greater risk for a rare type of vaginal and cervical cancer. A woman whose mother took DES should tell her doctor about her exposure and have pelvic exams done by a doctor familiar with conditions related to DES.

Women who took DES during pregnancy may themselves have a slightly higher risk for developing breast cancer. Again, they should tell their doctors about their exposure. At this time, there does not appear to be an increased risk of breast cancer for daughters who were exposed to DES before birth. However, more studies are needed to follow these daughters as they age and enter the age range when breast cancer is more common.

Finally, there is evidence that DES-exposed sons may have testicular abnormalities, such as undescended or abnormally small testicles. The possible risk for testicular cancer in these men is under study.

Family Trends. Does cancer run in families? Certain types of cancer—including melanoma and cancers of the breast, ovary, prostate, and colon—do tend to occur more often in some families than in the rest of the population. It's often unclear, however, whether a pattern of cancer in a given family is due primarily to heredity, to factors in the family's environment or lifestyle, or to chance, pure and simple.

Researchers have learned that cancer is caused by changes (called *mutations* or *alterations*) in the genes that control the normal growth and death of cells. Most cancer-causing gene mutations are the result of factors in an individual's lifestyle or environment. However, some are inherited; that is, they are passed from parent to child. Having such an inherited gene alteration does not mean that someone is certain to develop cancer; rather, it means that his or her risk for cancer is increased.

HOW IS CANCER TREATED?

Traditionally, a limited number of cancer therapies have been used. The most common are surgery, chemotherapy, and radiation therapy, which may be used separately or in combination, depending on the nature of the diagnosis and the physician making it. Certainly, anyone who has been diagnosed with cancer should explore all the possible treatment options and consult other medical professionals, as well.

Surgery involves removing the cancerous tissue and perhaps some of the surrounding area. It's often the first line of treatment for cancers involving tumors, such as breast cancer and colon cancer. The basic premise is to cut out the bad tissue and leave the good. The problem is, in many cases, some bad tissue is unintentionally left behind, while in others, too much good tissue is removed. The consequences of removing too much or too little can be devastating and even fatal, depending on the area of the body. In removing a brain tumor, for instance, the room for error is not large. The accuracy of surgery to remove cancerous tissue will continue to improve with advances in both diagnostic and surgical techniques.

Surgery is often followed by another type of treatment in an effort to destroy any remaining cancer cells. One of the most common is *chemotherapy*, which involves administering a highly toxic drug through a series of treatments that may span a week's or even a month's time. The drugs used in chemotherapy, such as 5-flurouricil (5-FU), are thought to be more harmful to the cancer cells than to the other cells of the body. These drugs act at the level of DNA, causing it to malfunction and thus preventing the cells from dividing. This is critical to stopping the spread of cancer, since cancerous cells multiply in an uncontrolled manner.

However, chemotherapy has some drawbacks. One is that in addition to destroying the cancerous cells, the drugs also get into the healthy cells, which can make the patient very sick, depending on the number of treatments needed and over how long a timeframe. Common side-effects of chemotherapy include severe nausea, loss of healthy cells, and hair loss. In addition, the success rate of chemotherapy depends largely upon what stage the cancer is at. That is, the more advanced the cancer, the less the likelihood that it can be treated successfully.

Put simply, there are four stages of cancer, and they are ordered according to degree of severity (that is, 1 is least serious and 4 is most serious). The first three stages are usually treated with surgery followed by chemotherapy. For people with stage 1 cancer, the success rate of this treatment approach is 85 to 90 percent; for people with stage 2, the success rate is 70 to 80 percent; and for people with stage 3, the success rate is 60 to 70 percent. People with stage 4 cancer are considered untreatable, unfortunately.

A growing trend is to administer what's called a *chemotherapy "cocktail"*: a combination of drugs intended to deliver a powerful blow to the cancer. For instance, the triplet of docetaxel, doxorubicin, and cyclophosphamide (TAC) has been found effective in treating node-positive breast cancer. In a recent three-year study by the Breast Cancer International Research Group (BCIRG), disease-free survival was significantly higher in patients who underwent the "cocktail" treatment rather than the regular chemotherapy regimen.

The third major cancer therapy is *radiotherapy* (or *radiation therapy*), in which a source of radiation is directed to the site of the cancer either with a stream or by a carrier molecule (often a protein called an *antibody*). Like chemotherapy, radiotherapy often follows surgery as a second line of defense. And again, more than one treatment may be needed across a timeframe of weeks or months, depending on the nature of the cancer. In some cases, treatment may be extended or restarted to deal with a possible recurrence of the cancer.

Radiotherapy isn't 100 percent effective in killing the cancerous cells. Plus, a common side-effect of radiotherapy is that good tissue is damaged, perhaps leading to future illness. As mentioned earlier, before having radiotherapy, a patient should talk with his or her doctor about the side-effects of radiation treatment, which may include increasing the risk of getting a second cancer.

A relatively new mode of cancer treatment is *laser ablation*, which involves blasting the cancer cells with a laser. There are several problems with this method. For instance, it's likely that not all of the cancer cells will be killed with one treatment, which will mean having to repeat the procedure. It's also possible that too much tissue will be killed or even that parts of the body will be destroyed. Given the newness of this technology, it's likely that these problems will lessen with development in laser and computer technology.

WHAT IS THE PROBIOTIC SOLUTION?

The body has a limited number of cells. If one dies, it's replaced with an exact copy of itself in the exact location. The whole body works like that. What happens in cancer is that the cells start to grow uncontrollably, which, by itself, is not bad. The problem is that in addition to growing, they do a number of harmful things: release toxins, disrupt the normal functioning of whatever tissues or organs they happen to be in, and consume a lot of energy.

What causes cancer cells to grow uncontrollably is the mutations that occur at the gene level, and those mutations can occur for several reasons. First, the cells may be attacked by something like a virus, which will attach itself to the normal human cell and then inject its DNA (or genetic material) into the DNA of the normal cell. This can (but does not always) disrupt the normal functioning of the otherwise healthy cell, causing mutation.

Alternatively, the mutations can occur as a result of exposure to *mutagenic compounds*, which are simply chemicals or substances that cause DNA to change. To understand this, think of each individual cell's DNA as being made up of four small letters—G, A, T, and C—that are organized in a precise way, such as GATCCCAAG. A single, small piece of DNA will always look just like that, even after the cell divides. That's how the DNA (sometimes called the *genetic code*) is passed on from generation to generation. But if, say, the T is changed to a C by something that causes mutation, then the code will read GACCCCAAG. This tiny change could make the difference in whether that cell lives or dies.

How does a mutation happen? Well, everything a cell does—*everything*—is the result of what its DNA says—or to use our example, by how the letters are arranged. Certain compounds can actually come in and change those letters. Those compounds are what are collectively referred to as *mutagens* or *carcinogens*. (There is a minor difference between the two, but it isn't relevant to this discussion.)

When DNA is doing its job, the cell is happy and normal. It divides a limited number of times, and given that, it dies at a predetermined time. All normal cells do this. But as part of this normal functioning—for instance, in replication/duplication—the DNA of the cell has to be "unwrapped," so to speak. (Most DNA is kept tightly packed for a number of reasons, one of which is that the stuff that does the packing actually protects the DNA from carcinogens.)

This unwrapping increases the chance of a bad compound attacking the DNA. The more often the DNA is unwrapped, the more likely it will be attacked and hurt. How well or how poorly it survives depends directly on the sequence of those four letters, which, in turn, can be affected by toxic, mutagenic, and carcinogenic compounds.

So, where do probiotics come in? They actually function in a number of ways. First, they can make substances that will interact with the offensive materials and detoxify them. Second, probiotics can actually take in the toxic materials and process them by various pathways, making them less toxic. Third, probiotics can physically keep out bad bacteria. This is good not just because bad bacteria, such as the infamous *E. coli* (which is often the culprit in cases of contaminated meat), can produce substances that make us feel sick and can even kill us but also because those same bad bacteria can take what would otherwise be innocuous materials and turn them into carcinogens.

Probiotics do this by physically displacing the bad bacteria. Inside the human gut, there is limited space. In order for a bacteria, either good or bad, to exert an effect on the health of the human host, it has to spend a little time hanging out—quite literally, in fact. That is, the bacteria must attach itself to the lining of the gastrointestinal (GI) tract in a process called *bacteria adherence*. Certain bacteria occupy certain areas of the GI tract. For instance, *Lactobacilli* tend to inhabit the upper portion, known as the *small intestine*, and *Bifidobacteria* tend to inhabit the colon, which is part of the *large intestine*.

Probiotics normally live and die just like human cells. As they age, they can be mutated so they do not bind as well. When that happens, there is an increased chance that any bad bacteria that are passing by might adhere in place of the probiotics as they start to lose their foothold on the intestinal lining. When the bad bacteria are established where they should not be, they can do a few things—none of them good.

First, these bacteria can chew away at the lining of the intestine. This means that the cells in the lining will have to be replaced, requiring the DNA to be unwrapped and thus increasing the chances of mutagenesis. Second, the bad bacteria can produce toxic compounds that will destroy the good bacteria and the human cells. Again, the human cells will try to replace themselves and have to divide again. (Clearly, because cells only have a limited number of lives, it's not good for them to have to replace themselves constantly.)

Third, the bad bacteria can take potentially noxious substances and make them very carcinogenic. Those carcinogens will then go on to wreak havoc in the normal cells as they try to go about their lives. Actually, the bad bacteria also do something the good bacteria do, but they do it in the opposite way. Both good and bad bacteria condition their environment; for instance, they can alter things such as the pH by secreting or not secreting acids. They can also produce bactericidal compounds that will kill off the opposite type of bacteria, good or bad. So, when the bad bacteria do this, there will be more and more bad guys around, causing trouble.

One solution to this problem is to add more good bacteria, which can be done by supplementing with probiotics. This might not be as simple as it sounds, as there are over 400 species (or types) of probiotics in the normal GI tract. To help sort things out, a number of companies have come up with what they believe are the most predominant bacteria normally found in healthy people. Typically, the list includes 10 to 20 different probiotics.

To give you an idea of what's out there on the market, let me mention the products of some of the larger suppliers I know and trust. For instance, MAK Wood carries *Bifobacterium-BB12, Bifidobacterium bifidum, B. infantis, B. lactis, B. animalis, B. longum, Lactobacillus (L.) acidophilus, LA-5 (L. acidophilus), L. bulgaricus, Streptococcus thermophilus, L. casei, L. paracasei, L. plantarum, L. rhamnosus, L. lactis, L. paracasei ssp. paracasei CRL-43,* and *Streptococcus thermophilus.* (In addition, MAK Wood qualifies the integrity of all their ingredients, including probiotics, using the MAKTech process, a highly technical and sophisticated quality control method. See Chapter 10 for more information on this.) The Danish company CHR Hansen carries *Bifidobacterium animalis (prev. lactis or bifidum) BB-12, B. longum, B. infantis, L. acidophilus LA-5, L. brevis, L. bulgaricus (Probio-Tec), L. paracasei ssp. paracasei CRL-431, L. plantarum, L. rhamnosus, L. salivarius, Lactococcus lactis,* and S. *thermophilus.* The French company Rhodia carries *Bifidobacterium bifidum, B. infantis, B. lactis, B. animalis, B. longum, L. acidophilus, L. bulgariucus, L. casei, L. paracasei, L. plantarum, L. rhamnosus, L. lactis,* and *Streptococcus thermophilus.*

While research on probiotics goes back over 100 years, the techniques required to mass produce and test probiotics have only been available for about 20 years. That's why, in large part, so few types of probiotics are available—only a couple dozen strains. The other reason for this scarcity has to do with the marketing of these products. Consider that most companies want to sell you their own wonderful probiotics, and in order to do that, they must show you how many studies have been done on their strains. Having limited amounts of funds available for research, companies focus on certain strains, rather than test all of them individually. The marketing gurus realize that you, the consumer, will be more impressed to see that 100 clinical studies have been done on a specific strain, such as *LA-5* or *BB-12* (even though they are all amazingly similar), than you will be to see that 100 different studies have been done on 100 different bugs (most of which are not available anyway).

Taking probiotics is not a one-time fix. To be sure, the toxic and potentially toxic compounds and bad bacteria in your body never stop coming. You must keep adding good bacteria to hold off the onslaught of bad bacteria. Also, the good bacteria will be under constant assault, and they can suffer mutations the same way normal cells do. When that happens, the cells will end up weakened or dead.

When the *probiotics* are weakened or dead, they cannot detoxify the noxious compounds and fend off the bad guys. The result is that the bad guys will eventually win. That's why you need to continually supplement your diet with new, fresh, viable probiotics. Make sure that fresh troops are constantly on guard, protecting your health.

We have made great strides in understanding cancer in all of its facets and guises. And along with these gains has come an increased survival rate. For instance, melanoma is now almost 100 percent curable, if caught early on. Ongoing research on other types of cancer will hopefully bring more of the same good news. The more we learn about the causes of cancer, the better we will be able to fight it—in fact, the better we will be able to prevent it!

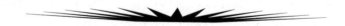

CHAPTER 2

A Recent Breakthrough—Why Probiotics Can Be the Magic Bullet against Coronary Heart Disease

WHAT IS CORONARY HEART DISEASE?

Coronary heart disease (CHD) is caused by a narrowing of the coronary arteries that feed the heart. It's the most common form of heart disease, affecting some 7 million Americans, and it's also the number-one killer of both men and women. Each year, more than 500,000 Americans die of heart attacks caused by CHD.

Many of these deaths could be prevented because CHD is related to certain aspects of lifestyle. Some of the *risk factors* for CHD, or things that increase your risk of developing the disease, are high blood pressure, high blood cholesterol, smoking, obesity, physical inactivity, diabetes, and stress—all of which can be controlled. On average, having high blood pressure, having high blood cholesterol, *or* being a smoker doubles your chance of developing heart disease. Therefore, a person who has all three of these risk factors is eight times more likely to develop heart disease than someone who has none. Also consider that being overweight increases the likelihood of developing high blood cholesterol and high blood pressure, and being physically inactive increases the risk of heart attack.

Other risk factors for CHD *cannot* be controlled, such as heredity, age, and sex. Heredity involves several issues, one of which is race/ethnicity. African Americans are more likely than European Americans to have severely high blood pressure and thus a higher risk of developing CHD. The risk for CHD is also higher among Mexican Americans, American Indians, native Hawaiians, and some Asian Americans. This elevated risk is partly due to higher rates of obesity and diabetes among these racial/ethnic groups. Other familial traits also put people at greater for CHD. For instance, most people with a strong family history of heart disease have one or more other risk factors, as well, such as high blood pressure or high cholesterol. For all these reasons, the children of parents with CHD are more likely to develop it themselves. This trend underscores the importance of addressing those risk factors for CHD that *can* be controlled, say, through lifestyle.

Age and sex are other risk factors that can't be controlled. As will be discussed later, CHD develops over time, which means the risk increases as someone ages. Four out of five people who die of CHD are 65 or older. Older women, especially, are more likely than men to die within a few weeks after having a heart attack. Even so, men are at greater risk for having a heart attack than are women, and men typically have a heart attack earlier in life. Even later in life, when the death rate from CHD among women increases dramatically, it's still lower than the death rate among men.

The relationship between sex and heart disease has been the focus of recent news stories, which have reported that women with CHD are often misdiagnosed. The reason behind this is that most of the models of heart disease have come from studying male anatomy and physiology and how *males* respond to diseases and to curative drugs. The problem is that men and women respond differently to diseases. Also, women are much more likely than men to get medical attention right away when they feel that something's wrong. Of course, getting an early diagnosis won't help if that diagnosis is wrong!

All of these factors increase your risk of developing CHD, but they do not describe all the causes of coronary heart disease. Even with none of these risk factors, you might still develop CHD. And while medical treatments for heart disease have come a long way, controlling the risk factors remains the most successful approach to preventing illness and death from CHD. In particular, getting regular exercise, eating a nutritious diet, and not smoking are the keys to controlling the risk factors for CHD.

WHAT CAUSES CORONARY HEART DISEASE?

To understand what causes CHD, you need to understand how the heart works. Like any muscle, the heart needs a constant supply of oxygen and nutrients, and these elements are carried to the heart by the blood in the coronary arteries. When the coronary arteries become narrowed or clogged, they cannot supply enough blood to the heart, which can have several effects.

If too little oxygen-carrying blood reaches the heart, it may respond with pain, which is called *angina*. This pain is usually felt in the chest or sometimes in the left arm and shoulder. However, the same inadequate blood supply may cause no symptoms, a condition called *silent angina*. When the blood supply is cut off completely, the result is a *heart attack*. When this occurs, the part of the heart that does not receive oxygen begins to die, and some of the heart muscle may be permanently damaged.

The thickening that occurs on the inside walls of the coronary arteries is called *atherosclerosis*, and it usually occurs when a person has high levels of *cholesterol*, a fat-like substance, in the blood. While circulating in the blood, cholesterol and fat build up on the walls of the arteries, making them more narrow and slowing or even blocking the flow of blood. When the level of cholesterol in the blood is high, there is a greater chance that it will be deposited onto the artery walls. This process begins in most people during their childhood and teenage years and gets worse as they get older.

What is *cholesterol*? Cholesterol, simply put, is nothing more than a molecule that the body uses as a building block to produce other types of compounds. Granted, this definition holds true for a lot of things, but it's sufficient for our discussion here. In fact, picturing cholesterol as a child's block or a Lego will be useful.

We hear a lot of talk about the different types of cholesterol, and a number of abbreviations are thrown around, such as *HDL (high-density lipoprotein), LDL (low-density lipoprotein),* and *HDL/LDL* (which is simply the ratio of the two). This is all a lot easier than it sounds. What's important to remember is that the HDLs are the good cholesterol and the LDLs are the bad cholesterol. The bad ones are those that will clog up your arteries, making them hard and constricted.

That is really the crux of the problem. Once flexibility is lost in the arteries, the blood pressure goes up and the optimal levels of blood and other nutrients cannot reach the various parts of the body—including the hardest working muscle of the body, the heart.

The earliest signs of CHD are often chest pain and shortness of breath. A person may feel heaviness, tightness, pain, burning, pressure, or squeezing in the chest, usually behind the breastbone but sometimes also in the arms, neck, or jaw. These are the signs that typically bring a patient to the doctor for the first time. However, some people never have any of these symptoms and only discover that they have CHD after they have had a heart attack. Women, especially, may be unfamiliar with the signs of CHD that are unique to women and may be unaware of their condition until they have had a heart attack.

It's important to know that the symptoms of CHD cover a wide range of severity. Some people have no symptoms at all, some have mild and intermittent chest pain, and some have more pronounced and steady pain. Still others have such severe symptoms of CHD that doing normal, everyday activities becomes difficult.

HOW IS CORONARY HEART DISEASE TREATED?

CHD is treated in a number of ways, depending on the seriousness of the disease. For many people, CHD can be managed by making lifestyle changes and taking medications. People with severe CHD may need surgery. In any case, once CHD develops, it requires lifelong management.

Lifestyle Changes

As noted earlier, despite advances in treating CHD, making lifestyle changes remains the single most effective way to stop the disease from progressing. In particular, the person with CHD needs to eat a lowfat diet, get regular exercise, and not smoke.

Changing your diet to one that is low in fat, especially saturated fat, and low in cholesterol will help reduce your level of blood cholesterol, a primary cause of atherosclerosis. In fact, it's even more important to keep blood cholesterol low *after* having a heart attack in order to help lower the risk of having another one. Eating less fat should also help you lose weight, and if you are overweight, losing weight can help lower your blood cholesterol. Losing weight is also the most effective lifestyle change you can make to reduce high blood pressure, another risk factor for atherosclerosis and heart disease.

People with CHD can also benefit from exercise. Recent research has shown that even moderate amounts of physical activity are associated with lower death rates from CHD. However, people with severe CHD may have to restrict their exercise somewhat. If you have CHD, check with your doctor to find out what kinds of exercise are best for you.

Smoking is one of the three major risk factors for CHD, so quitting smoking is a major lifestyle change in terms of preventing heart disease. Quitting smoking dramatically lowers the risk of having a heart attack and also reduces the risk of having a second heart attack in people who have already had one.

Medications

If making lifestyle changes was enough to prevent or control CHD, then medications would never be used. Diet changes, in particular, have been the traditional remedy for bad or high cholesterol, and while diet can make a difference, it doesn't always take care of the situation. The body has the ability to produce its own cholesterol and to do that in rather high amounts when needed. This is a problem for someone who's trying to control his or her cholesterol level by diet modification alone.

To help solve this problem, scientists have looked into ways to modify the body's ability to produce cholesterol. The result has been a class of drugs known as *statins*, which generally address cholesterol synthesis by attacking the pathway at some point. Unfortunately, statins tend to be nondiscriminant and knock out cholesterol production without regard for the type of cholesterol and the fact that the body does need some. Without some cholesterol, you would probably die. For instance, one type of statin, called *Lovastatin*, knocks out HMG-CoA reductase, an enzyme that is necessary for the production of cholesterol. Some of these pharmaceutical drugs also carry unwanted side-effects, such as muscle pain, tenderness, or weakness (especially associated with fever and a general feeling of discomfort); rash; yellow skin or eyes; unusual bleeding or bruising; swelling of the hands, face, lips, eyes, throat, or tongue; difficulty swallowing or breathing; and sore throat or hoarseness.

Some natural products are very similar to the pharmaceutical cholesterol-controlling drugs. These products are sold over the counter, mainly in health-food stores but sometimes in large discount retailers, as well. One such example is *Red Rice Yeast (RRY)*, or as it's also called, *Red Yeast Rice*. It naturally contains high levels of the same compound that is found in some of the pharmaceutical drugs to control cholesterol. RRY has been used for thousands of years in traditional Chinese medicine for this exact purpose, and Western science is now beginning to catch up.

Other medications are prescribed according to the nature of the patient's CHD and other health issues. The symptoms of angina can generally be controlled by any of several types of drugs, such as *beta-*

blockers, which decrease the workload on the heart, and *nitroglycerine* (along with other nitrates) and *calcium-channel blockers*, which relax the arteries. In addition, aspirin and other platelet-inhibitory and anticoagulant drugs can be used to thin the blood and prevent the tendency to form clots.

Beta-blockers are typically given to people who have had a heart attack in order to decrease the likelihood of their having another one. People with elevated blood cholesterol that is unresponsive to treatment through dietary and weight-loss measures may be prescribed cholesterol-lowering drugs, such as lovastatin, colestipol, cholestyramine, gemfibrozil, and niacin. Someone with impaired pumping of the heart may be treated with digitalis drugs or ACE (angiotension converting enzyme) inhibitors. And when high blood pressure or fluid retention is present, this condition is also treated.

If you have CHD, ask your doctor which medications you are taking, what they do, and what side-effects are common. Knowing more about these things will help you stick to the schedule that has been prescribed for you.

Surgery

Not all individuals can control CHD with lifestyle changes and medication. Surgery may be recommended for those who continue to have frequent or disabling angina despite the use of medications and for those who have severe blockage of one or more coronary arteries.

The first type of surgery, called *coronary angioplasty* or *balloon angioplasty*, involves inserting a catheter with a tiny balloon at its tip into a narrowed (clogged) coronary artery. The balloon is then inflated and deflated to stretch or break open the narrowed passage and improve the bloodflow. The balloon-tipped catheter is then removed. Strictly speaking, angioplasty is not surgery. It's done while the patient is awake and may last one to two hours.

If angioplasty doesn't widen the artery or if complications occur, a *coronary bypass operation* may be needed. In this type of surgery, a blood vessel, usually taken from the leg or chest, is grafted onto the blocked coronary artery, bypassing the blocked area. If more than one artery is blocked, a bypass can be done on each. The blood can then go around the obstruction to supply the heart with enough blood to relieve the patient's chest pain.

Having bypass surgery relieves the symptoms of heart disease but does not cure it. And in most cases, the patient still has to make a number of lifestyle changes after the operation. If his or her normal lifestyle includes smoking, eating a high-fat diet, or getting no exercise, changes will be definitely advised.

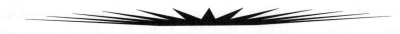

WHAT IS THE PROBIOTIC SOLUTION?

Taking probiotics has only recently been considered as a means of controlling cholesterol. Why only recently? There has been anecdotal evidence for many years of the correlation between taking probiotics and having low cholesterol. Consuming fermented foods, such as yogurt, and even plain probiotics was known to help lower cholesterol, so scientists set out to study that.

What they found in the probiotic studies on cholesterol was that when very high doses were used—well over 100 billion live organisms per dose—there was a reduction in blood cholesterol. Even more important, an increase in the ratio of HDL to LDL was observed. And the higher the HDL compared to the LDL, the higher the ratio.

Why is this important? If the LDLs are clogging things up, think of the HDLs as cleaning things out. As mentioned earlier, think of the LDLs as being like little Legos, with connectors that allow multiple cholesterol molecules to bind to each other. The LDLs collect in the arteries and build on one another, slowly clogging things up. The HDLs, on the other hand, are like Legos without connectors. Also, since the HDLs can't bind to other things, they have a kind of "bowling ball" effect and knock out the LDLs from wherever they are grouping. So, if there are many more HDLs in comparison to LDLs, then fewer LDLs will be able to build up. Remember, the HDLs and the LDLs *combine* (numerically, not physically) to form the number that's called *total cholesterol*. It's all rather simple.

Given these benefits, probiotics have been looked at and used in high concentration. Strains such as *Lactobacillus acidophilus (LA)* have been used in 10s to 100s of billions per dose, and reductions in total blood cholesterol have been observed. More recently, some other specific strains have been looked at, such as *Lactobacillus reuteri (LR)*, and the findings have been very important and interesting. In contrast to some of the other probiotics, *LR* can be used at very low levels to achieve very significant levels of cholesterol reduction. This is big news! Bear in mind, specific strains have been used for these studies, which will be discussed in more detail later in this section. But for now, remember that you want to find a strain that has scientific backing in terms of how it was chosen for production.

In order for the probiotics to function well in cholesterol reduction, it seems that they need to survive being ingested into the intestines. Now, why is that? When you eat probiotics, they enter your stomach and if they are not resistant to the acid, they will be destroyed by it. In fact, the vast majority will be killed. Then, when the survivors reach your intestines, they come in contact with another very harsh substance called *bile*, and they take another hit. Among its other functions, bile also serves as an antimicrobial substance. So, if the probiotics are not resistant to acid or bile, then they will not survive long enough to be of benefit.

How do those probiotics that survive help reduce cholesterol? As mentioned earlier, the body normally produces its own cholesterol; it doesn't get it just from the diet. That's why dietary modification is not always successful and when it is, the success is marginal at best. The body produces cholesterol and does a number of things with it. Again, think of cholesterol as a building block or Lego. One of the things the body builds with cholesterol is bile. Bile is produced in the liver, stored in the gall bladder, and secreted into the intestines to assist with digestion. The primary job of bile is to emulsify fat, which is a fancy way of saying it assists in the digestion of fat. After that, bile gets reabsorbed into the intestines and finds its way back to the gall bladder, where it's stored until it's needed again.

The body has evolved to be very efficient, and it doesn't like to waste energy. Keep in mind, it takes energy to make compounds such as cholesterol and bile from scratch. It's much easier just to reabsorb what has already been made. The body does this with enzymes, water, bile, and so on. The body likes to recycle as much as it can. It's the ultimate conservationist!

Bile can suffer two fates when it reaches the intestines after being secreted from the gall bladder: It can either go on to do its job (that is, to assist in digesting fat), or it can be broken down by a process called *deconjugation*. How this happens is not important. What is important is that the gastrointestinal microflora can have an effect on the deconjugation of bile. If the bile is deconjugated, then there is a greater chance it will be flushed out of the body with other waste materials. There will still be some reabsorption, but it will be minimal.

If the bile gets excreted, it will obviously not be reabsorbed and recycled back to the gall bladder. The gall bladder needs to maintain a certain level of bile, and it will do whatever it has to do to maintain that level. As noted earlier, bile is produced in the liver from cholesterol. If the bile level drops because of lack of circulation back into the gall bladder—which, in turn, is a result of probiotics acting on the bile in the intestines—then the body will have to produce more. The liver will sense that the level of bile has dropped and respond automatically by making more.

The net result is that the body will start drawing on its cholesterol reserves in order to make more bile. The body will start feeding on itself, which is a good thing, at least in this case. Cholesterol will literally be pulled out of the blood and used by the liver to produce bile. This has a very pronounced and measurable effect.

We see a good result when high doses of probiotics are used. We also see a good result when low doses of some of the more acid- and bile-resistant organisms are used. *LR* has been shown to be very acid and bile resistant. It can survive the journey into the intestines, where it can start pumping away on the bile and deconjugating it, resulting in the excretion of the bile. *LR* has been observed to produce a 38 percent decrease in total cholesterol.

This is stunning, given the so-called *one-to-two rule*, which states that a 1 percent reduction of blood cholesterol causes a 2 percent lower risk of coronary heart disease. Remember, we're talking about a 38 percent reduction in cholesterol here, so that means that taking *LR* probiotics can give you at least a 76 percent lower risk of CHD. That is major!

These beneficial effects can be achieved not only by taking high levels of probiotics but also by taking lower levels of some select strains. There are probably many different variants of each strain, each more or less acid and bile tolerant. What you should look for are products that use strains selected by the best technology available, such as DNA fingerprinting and cell-wall structure analysis.

Some companies have lines of products in which high-quality selection criteria are met. MAKTech is one such line, and I am sure there are others. (See the Resources section at the end of this book.) I know the MAKTech line has actually taken this step further and isolated the components of probiotics that are beneficial. In the case of cholesterol reduction, there is an enzyme called a *hydrolase* that is responsible for the deconjugation of bile. The MAKTech line offers this enzyme for people who don't want to take probiotics, for whatever reason—say, due to allergies. This sort of product offers these individuals all the advantages plus some extra choices.

Anyone who is concerned about getting CHD will want to take probiotics, even if he or she doesn't care about all the other ailments discussed in this book. Taking probiotics as part of a healthy diet has been proven to have positive effects on CHD and other related conditions.

CHD is something we all need to be aware of. Women, in particular, should make sure they find a physician who understands women's health issues, including their special risks for CHD.

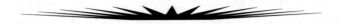

CHAPTER 3

Why Probiotic Therapy Offers New Hope for Autism

WHAT IS AUTISM?

Autism is classified as one of the pervasive developmental disorders of the brain. As such, it's not a disease but rather a disorder.

How prevalent is this disorder? Estimates of the incidence of autism in the general population vary greatly, depending on the diagnostic criteria used. Some estimates show that autism affects as few as 5 of every 10,000 people, but others put the incidence as high as 1 in 80. In reality, the incidence of autism may be several times higher than previously thought. Autism strikes males four times more often than females.

People with classical autism have three types of symptoms: impaired social interaction, problems with verbal and nonverbal communication, and unusual or severely limited activities and interests. More specifically, people with autism may be self-absorbed and unable to interact socially; they may also have behavior problems and language dysfunction (such as *echolalia*). These symptoms can vary in severity. In addition, people with autism often have abnormal responses to sound, touch, and other sensory stimulation.

The symptoms of autism usually appear during the first three years of childhood and continue through life. In many children, the symptoms improve with intervention or with age. Some people with autism eventually lead normal or near-normal lives. However, the onset of adolescence can worsen behavior problems in some children, and parents should be ready to adjust treatment for the child's changing needs.

The accumulated symptoms of autism are sometimes categorized as *autism spectrum disorders*, or ASD. This categorization fits with theories suggesting that people with autism have several maladies. About one-third of the children with ASD eventually develop epilepsy. This risk is highest in those with severe cognitive impairment and motor deficits.

Despite this range of symptoms, people with autism have a normal life expectancy.

WHAT CAUSES AUTISM?

While the exact cause of autism remains elusive, considerable advances have been made in recent years. These advances have come from study of the geographic localization, biological, and psychological aspects of the disease. From these studies, several theories have emerged.

One theory is that some people have a genetic predisposition to autism; researchers are looking for clues about which genes contribute to this increased susceptibility. Other studies of people with autism have found abnormalities in several regions of the brain, which suggests that autism results from a disruption of early fetal brain development. In some children, environmental factors also may play a role. Additionally, due to the timeframe of when the disease is initially observed (that is, in infancy), there has been an association between autism and childhood vaccination.

Other theories point to diet as playing a major role in the development of autism. It's thought that opioid-type peptides (or exorphins) are produced due to maldigestion of casein and gluten. Casein and gluten are proteins commonly found in dairy and wheat, respectively. (This will be discussed in more detail in the final section of this chapter.)

Several previous notions about the nature and causes of autism have been disproved. For instance, it was once commonly believed that autism resulted from a lack of parental affection, and mothers, in particular, were blamed for being cold toward their children. (They were sometimes referred to by the medical profession as "refrigerator mothers.") As silly as it sounds, this theory went unquestioned, at least publicly, until about 1970. Another popular theory about the so-called savant tendencies of autistics was popularized by the mass media through such movies as *Rain Man*. While it's true that some individuals with autism have amazing abilities in certain areas—such as recognizing and repeating strings of numbers and music and having extraordinary artistic abilities—no clear relationship has been established between these skills and autism.

HOW IS AUTISM TREATED?

There is currently no cure for autism, but appropriate treatment may bring about relatively normal development and reduce undesirable behaviors. Different types of therapies are designed to remedy specific symptoms. For instance, educational/behavioral therapies emphasize highly structured and often intensive skill-oriented training. Doctors also may prescribe a variety of drugs to reduce symptoms of autism. Other interventions are available, but few, if any, scientific studies support their use.

The prevailing nutritional therapies attempt to remedy autism in three ways, used either singly or in combination: diet restriction (avoiding dairy and wheat), supplementation with exogenous enzymes, and supplementation with probiotic bacteria. Until recently, none of the therapies addressed the molecular mechanisms that may be at work in the development and progression of autism.

The following section will look at the molecular and cellular mechanisms that are possibly related to autism and discuss how they can be used to treat the disease through the use of various nutrients. The link between autism and unusual immune and inflammatory responses will also be explored in the context of probiotics.

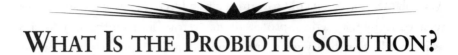

WHAT IS THE PROBIOTIC SOLUTION?

Pioneers in the field of autism first observed the significant correlation between the symptoms of autism and an impaired ability to adequately digest peptides/proteins from dairy (casein) and wheat (gluten). During digestion, preopioid-type compounds in the diet, typically from casein and gluten, seem to be activated due to an incomplete breakdown of proteins. These partial proteins or peptides, which are called *exorphins* (that is, casomorphins and gluteomorphins or gliadorphin), are then easily transferred across the lumen of the gut into the bloodstream; they are carried to the brain, where they exert an opioid-type action.

The transfer of peptides across the lumen of the gut is thought to occur at a high level in someone with autism because of the leaky nature of his or her gastrointestinal (GI) tract. According to the *exorphin theory* of autism, the attenuated level of a gut enzyme called *Dipeptididyl-peptidase IV (DPPIV)* could manifest as autistic symptoms. DPPIV is one of the enzymes that specifically digests exorphins so they don't interact with the body's own natural neural signaling.

Ingesting probiotics can help repair this leaky gut by providing a physical barrier that prevents bad bacteria (or *pathogens*) from attaching to and then moving across from the lumen to the inside of the body and causing *bacteremia* (or bacteria in the blood). Not only do the probiotics physically keep the bad bacteria at bay, but they also allow the body to recover from the physical distress those bacteria can cause. This allows the body to heal itself, to a large extent. In short, ingesting probiotics helps repair the GI tract of the autistic individual.

Another level at which probiotics are functional and beneficial to people with autism goes back to the exorphins in the diet. Recently, my own lab published findings on the use of enzymes and probiotics in the treatment of autism. A distinction was made between the two, but in reality, the line between probiotics and enzymes is not that clearcut—at least, not for a discussion of autism. The reason is that the probiotics contain very high levels of a variety of enzymes, several of which may be important for people with autism.

While other studies have been undertaken on the use of enzymes to treat autism, none have been reported in the literature at this time. And while my lab's study is similar to these others in structure, we used a unique enzyme formulation. In addition to adding several new enzymes, my lab's study is the first to report the therapeutic potential of *genomeceuticals*, which are designed to stimulate the body's own production of both the DPPIV enzyme and probiotics.

An important element of that formula is *galactose*, which is a simple sugar. It's almost identical to *glucose*, but the body doesn't use it in the same way. Galactose is believed to function at two levels. The first is as a genomeceutical, in which it is believed to increase the gut expression of the DPPIV gene present in the body. This allows for a greater level of DPPIV enzyme in the enterocytes (gut cells), promoting the more thorough breakdown of any exorphins produced by the proteases. The second and equally interesting possibility is that galactose serves as a fuel source of the beneficial microflora (that is, probiotics) in the gut. This is important because the probiotic organisms themselves contain enzymes capable of breaking down such exorphins.

Research has shown that the probiotic organisms currently used as health supplements contain analogues of the DPPIV enzyme (for example, PepX), which is known to be able to digest exorphins. With over 10 trillion microorganisms in the gut, their contribution of enzymatic activity can far exceed that of the enterocytes. It is well documented that galactose is a *prebiotic* (that is, it stimulates the growth of probiotics) and can therefore increase the number of probiotics in the gut.

Thus, it seems that increases occur both in the level of DPPIV in the gut and in the level of DPPIV-type activity (contributed by a large increase in the bacterial flora). And due to the rapid formation of any exorphins from the high level of acid stable protease, the result is that the levels of absorbed exorphins drops below the threshold required for manifestation of the parameters measured. To test this hypothesis, future studies are planned to assay urinary polypeptide levels on retained samples both before and after treatment. Future studies will also look at blood peptide levels both before and after treatment. Additionally, research is planned to determine how genomeceuticals contribute to the formula. Again, increasing levels of galactose will be assessed against all the parameters measured in the present study, along with blood levels of exorphins and stool levels of various probiotic species.

The only known contraindication for the use of galactose is in a fairly rare metabolic disorder called *galactosemia*. However, the amount of galactose in the formula (100 milligrams) is far less than the amount consumed in drinking a glass of milk. A typical glass of milk contains around 12 grams of lactose, which, when broken down, would contribute 6 grams of galactose to the diet—or approximately 60 times the amount in a single capsule of one of the products used.

As an uncontrolled pilot clinical study, work in my lab has had tremendous value in treating people with autism. The overwhelming majority of parameters measured show significant benefits from the enzyme blend, and very few negative reactions were associated with it. In addition, this is the first time a genomeceutical approach has been therapeutically applied—not just to autism but to any disorder. While the relationship between autism and ASDs still remains elusive, clearly, the present study advances the knowledge base for improving treatments.

One of the things that's observed in treating people with autism (and in a variety of other situations in which probiotics are used) is that over time, the same strain seems to have less and less positive effects on the body. Recently, I addressed this with the *Brudnak method* of pulsing and rotating probiotics, as I conceived of this theory and first wrote about it. (This is discussed in more detail later in this section and also in Chapter 10.)

Ten years ago, most probiotic products contained either *Lactobacillus acidophilus* or *Bifidobacterium lactis (bifidum)*. If someone was really lucky, he or she could find a combination of the two and possibly a couple of yogurt strains *(Lactobacillus bulgariucus)* thrown in. Many of these contained only a few 100 million viable cells at the time of manufacture. While that may sound like a lot of organisms, especially when we are conditioned to think of bacteria as being bad, current data show that those numbers were probably far too low to have done very much good. This was true at least in the short-term therapeutic application of probiotics.

What's changed in the past 10 years? As more and more data have come in, it has become apparent that at least 1 billion organisms per dose are needed to achieve any real clinical significance. In a recent study, 10 billion *Bifidobacterium* were given per day in milk and the immune markers were measured. A significant increase in phagocytic activity of granulocytes was observed.

Another study looked at the preventive effect that probiotics have in warding off infections in cancer patients. Thirty patients (35 episodes) were included. *Lactobacilli* were given as two capsules, three times a day for 30 days, starting at the initiation of the patient's chemotherapy. Each capsule contained a 50/50 mix of *Bifidobacterium lactis* and *Lactobacillus acidophilus*, 4 billion organisms per capsule. The occurrence of fever was significantly postponed from a median time of 8 days to 12 days. Clearly, probiotics can play an important role in treating even the most serious conditions, such as cancer.

The level of ammonia in the blood of people with autism is another research concern. The use of probiotics can easily assist with the reduction of circulating ammonia. One study used 5 billion organisms of either *B. lactis* or *B. breve* in caecal contents (or feces). In this study, researchers also observed a corresponding drop in the pH of the caecal contents. This lends support for the use of probiotics in detoxification protocols.

The whole area of detoxification of the body is very popular in the autism community. Doctors use things such as DMSA, EDTA, and other such *chelating agents*. (To *chelate* means to grab or surround something.)

Detoxification is relevant to treating autism because it has been suggested that environmentally acquired mercury—ingested through causal contact or through vaccination—is the culprit behind autism and ASDs.

An area related to detoxification but yet unexplored is the body's own endogenous enteric bacteria: probiotics. The rationale is that the gut associated lymphoid tissue (GALT) serves as a sort of lynchpin in the establishment and/or progression of autism. It's known that bacteria can detoxify methyl mercury (organic) using the *mer genes*. The mer genes are required to detoxify organic mercury compounds by converting them to volatile and much less toxic elemental mercury and inorgano-mercurials.

The mer genes are organized in a regulated operon, which may be genomically or extrachromosomally housed. The group of mer genes consists of *mer R*, which codes for Hg(II)-sensing, DNA-binding, regulatory protein; *mer A*, which codes for the mercuric-ion-reducing protein; and one or more of the genes *mer P*, *mer T*, and/or *mer C*, which code for proteins involved in moving the mercuric ions into the cytoplasm.

There is growing interest in the bacteria that harbor these genes, as they may be able to detoxify the body of mercury. This is a very hot topic now; in fact, it received a congressional review in April 2000. Since ordinary probiotics have been shown to detoxify mercury and have a long history of safe use, it seems a natural fit to use them to support proper functioning of the GALT, which is linked with immunity and overall health of a person.

Obviously, as the probiotics take up the mercury, more will be needed to replace those that pass through the system. The goal is not to provide constant circulation but rather to flush out the mercury in the probiotics along with the other waste. (See the Bibliography section [specifically, Brudnak 2002c] for a more detailed explanation of the system.)

Probiotic supplementation has been demonstrated to be safe and effective for a wide variety of conditions, including antibiotic side-effects, diarrhea and constipation, lactose malabsorption, and cholesterol reduction. Dosages ranging from 1 to almost 500 billion organisms have been used without complications. Current trends seem to indicate that a range of 10 to 100 billion live organisms is most effective in treating the variety of conditions just mentioned.

At least two different companies have high-dose products on the market, containing 20 and 30 billion organisms per capsule. Interestingly, both of these products were originally designed for use in different markets: people who are environmentally challenged and those who have autism (and Down syndrome), respectively. In terms of marketing, two conclusions seem obvious here: There is a need for high-dose probiotics to treat selective conditions, and there is also a need for a variety of products.

Thus, it seems that while a low-dose, run-of-the-mill *L. acidophilus* (providing it's well produced) can be great for a general maintenance program, often times, a much higher dose is needed to achieve clinical significance. Additionally, it's becoming more and more apparent that including other strains, such as *Lactobacillus rhamnosus* or *Lactobacillus plantarum* (an exciting up-and-coming star), can have a dramatic effect. The inclusion of multiple strains is beneficial for the specific conditions and may also play another important role in the application of probiotics.

I recently had a conversation with Dr. Stephanie G. Hoener, a naturopathic physician based in Portland, Oregon (see Resources for contact information). She specializes in assisting children with special needs, such as those with autism, and frequently speaks in the medical community on issues such as autism and detoxification. Dr. Hoener had this to say about using high-dose probiotics to treat children with autism:

> We often have to start patients on 20 to 60 billion organisms per day in order to get the beneficial effects. The majority of children with autism have severely compromised intestinal function and large numbers of pathogenic yeast and bacteria, so dosing this high is often what is needed in order to

begin the process of normalizing digestive function. Usually, we can dose even higher than this with even better results—as high as 100 billion organisms per day or higher, depending on the child's age. In addition to supporting GI function, these high doses of probiotics also help to strengthen these children's immune systems, which are often significantly compromised.

Increasingly, the use of mono- and bi-strain products brings reports of reductions in the clinical effects seen over time. For instance, in the case of autism, a child for whom pretreatment causes diarrhea or some other gastrointestinal distress will improve dramatically when first supplemented with these products. He or she will start producing well-formed stools on a regular basis. However, in some cases, the child will go back to the previous distressed state. Two approaches seem to have answers for this troubling phenomenon.

First is the "pulse" step of the Brudnak method of pulsing and rotating probiotics, mentioned earlier. Here, when the clinical effect begins to change, the physician can stop the probiotic supplementation for a period of time and then later repeat the application. The body appears to reset itself after the therapy has been stopped. During this period, changes occur in the GI tract that may make the local environment more hospitable to the probiotics. Additionally, there are certainly changes in the immune functioning of the gut.

It's well established that the intestines are a major source of immune competence. It's also well established that certain genetic elements respond to heavy metals—in particular, to mercury. Perhaps upon first being exposed to the probiotics, the gut-associated immune system is mobilized and attacks the probiotics. Then, after withdrawal of the probiotics, the immune reaction tapers off until another exposure occurs. This cycle is not a bad thing; in fact, it can be used to great advantage by pulsing with probiotics.

A variation on that theme also can be employed. It seems logical that instead of withdrawing all of the probiotics for any period of time, another product, containing different organisms, could be substituted. For instance, if a product that contains just *L. rhamnosus* is being used and the above condition presents, a product that contains just *Bifidobacterium* could be substituted in a subsequent treatment. If a single strain of *Bifidobacterium* is used and, again, the same situation occurs, then a third product containing several strains could be substituted. What strain is used in what instance would certainly have to be determined on a case-by-case basis, according to the physician's observations. In the foreseeable future, products will be designed specifically to address the issue in this way. This probiotic rotation will be applicable in a variety of situations.

Dr. Hoener also passed along a clinical observation regarding how the body becomes accustomed to one organism, such that it has less and less of a positive effect:

> In children with autism, it is extremely common to see that they do very well on a probiotic supplement for a period of time and then it appears to lose its efficacy. For example, after starting a probiotic, they may have a resolution of their diarrhea, more well-formed stools, less gassiness and abdominal bloating, and less abdominal discomfort. If these benefits appear to lessen after a period of several weeks, we can switch them to a different strain of probiotic and the positive improvements will generally return. I've spoken with dozens of parents who have tried this pulsing-and-rotating approach with their autistic child and obtained very favorable results.

Clearly, the area of probiotics is still in its infancy. This neonate will soon grow up, however, as major pharmaceutical companies enter this exciting and efficacious area of health care. As clinical data from the application of probiotics to conditions such as autism come to light, consumers' and patients' awareness of the importance of these organisms—and the demand for treatment using them—will likewise increase. With that, we can expect that better products, tailored to specific conditions, will also be developed.

Currently, there is a demand in the autism community for foods and supplements that are both casein and gluten free *(or GFCF)*. There is also an increasing demand for probiotic organisms. Some question has arisen about the ability to produce probiotic organisms that can qualify as GFCF. The GFCF issue presents several technical issues, which have not yet been addressed.

Today, the overwhelming majority of probiotics are produced in growth media that, at some point, contain at least one dairy product. However, it's generally agreed that by paying proper attention to growth conditions, as well as processing methods, the final products can be considered casein (or milk) free. This is because during normal growth and processing, the bacteria consume the dairy elements of the growth media and the residuals are separated during the concentration/ purification of the probiotics. However, there are often problems demonstrating this result due to the inherent problems of current *assay methods* (that is, the methods used to take apart the substance and examine its individual elements).

Several types of assay methods are currently used to detect casein in probiotics. The first is precipitation and quantification by total protein methods, such as the Kjeldahl procedure. The second is by an enzyme-linked immunosorbent assay (ELISA), which utilizes antibodies to detect the casein as a target antigen with subsequent reporter systems (for example, colorometric). Let's look at both in some detail.

The *total protein method* evolved out of the food-processing industry as a way to test milk products for casein. It relies on the fact that the vast majority of protein present in milk is casein, and for this industry, this method has proven useful. Additionally, the probiotics are living organisms that produce a wide variety of proteins. These, too, can contribute to a false-positive signal from the reporter system due to a similarity to casein in sequence. The chance of this happening when using a *monoclonal* antibody (mAb) is much less than when using a *polyclonal* antibody (pAb). However, the standard kit used to detect casein contains pAbs, not mAbs.

The technicalities of the antibodies and their differences are not important. What *is* important is that they give different results. In particular, different bacteria produce different levels of various proteins, so there can be seemingly inconsistent results from species to species and even strain to strain. Because probiotic organisms contain thousands of different proteins at any given time, the total protein method is not appropriate for determining casein in any given culture.

The second assay method—the *ELISA method*—also has several drawbacks. First, it's most desirable in this method to use a monoclonal antibody (mAb), not a polyclonal antibody (pAb), for reasons of specificity. With a mAb, the chance of getting a false-positive is much less because the mAb is considerably more specific for the desired target (in this case, casein) than is the pAb. The pAb is, by definition, specific for several, if not many, different targets. Why? A pAb is not one single antibody but consists of many different Abs—hence, the prefix *poly-*. For many purposes, a pAb is sufficient. The reasons for using a pAb over a mAb range from time to cost. In sum, a pAb can be produced much faster than a mAb and at much less cost.

The ELISA assay is a very good assay technique, but it's less than desirable for assaying casein in probiotics. The reason for this (in addition to those just mentioned) has to do with how the reporter portion of the ELISA functions. While there are different ways to perform the ELISA assay, they all can be generalized as follows: During ELISA, when a target molecule binds to the Ab, a subsequent enzymatic reaction (typically, the enzyme is linked to the antibody) is used to report that the binding occurred. This enzymatic reaction, more often than not, involves a peroxidase or phosphatase. Herein lies the problem, because probiotics produce peroxidases and phosphatases.

The problem is further confounded because different bacteria produce different levels of these enzymes. For instance, *Lactobacillus acidophilus (LA)* produces peroxidase. Not surprisingly, *LA* shows up as a positive using the ELISA method, even when produced using the very same procedure for other strains that show up as negatives. Furthermore, other enzymes are probably produced by the bacteria, which can similarly trigger the reporter system and result in a false-positive.

A third, although much less common, method for detecting casein utilizes *gel* (typically, SDS-polyacrylamide) *chromatography*. In this method, cellular extracts are placed in an electric field at one end of a gel matrix. The matrix allows the smaller proteins to move through first and the larger proteins to migrate more slowly—thus, lagging relative to the smaller proteins. This differential mobility in the gel affords a separation of proteins and protein fragments. The main problem with this method is that it is not only possible but probable that two very different proteins (based on sequence) can have the same mobility in the gel. This limitation can be overcome, to some degree, using isoelectric-focusing gels. This process also has similar problems associated with it.

Keep in mind that the fundamental reason for concern over casein is the fear of producing exorphins from it. This is important because the probiotic organisms that are being subjected to the casein analysis themselves contain enzymes that are capable of breaking down such exorphins. As noted earlier, research has recently shown that probiotic organisms currently utilized as health supplements contain analogues of the DPPIV enzyme (for example, PepX), which is known to be able to digest exorphins. Noteworthy is the fact that the higher the concentration of probiotics a supplement might contain, the higher the chance it will test as a false-positive for casein while concurrently producing unusually large amounts of the DPPIV analogues.

Taken as a whole, this information clarifies several standing issues regarding both probiotic supplementation in treating autism and reported test discrepancies. In light of recent advances in understanding about the underlying enzymology of probiotic organisms, it makes sense to view casein testing in light of the actual biological significance that any detected presence might have.

Further, the current state-of-the-art of casein testing should be given proper consideration. I buy my products from a manufacturer who has been selling probiotics specifically *for many years*, not just a few. Anyone who decides to go with a start-up company should make sure it's associated with a reputable manufacturer. It's important to look for quality trademarks, such as MAKTech and HOWARU. (See the Resources section at the end of the book for contact information.)

When I look for products for the autism community in my consulting work, I usually look for those from certain manufacturers. (Again, see the list of suppliers in the Resources section.) In addition to having good probiotic products and plans for future products that fit the Brudnak method of pulsing and rotating probiotics, they also carry food items that are casein and gluten free. Several of the companies I know are very helpful, and several seem especially interested in the autism community and its kids.

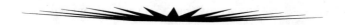

CHAPTER 4

Why Probiotics May Spell Relief for Alzheimer's Disease

WHAT IS ALZHEIMER'S DISEASE?

Alzheimer's disease (AD) is a progressive neurodegenerative disease characterized by deterioration in skills involving memory, language, visual/spatial perception, judgment, and attitude but preserved motor function. AD usually begins after age 65; however, its onset may occur as early as age 40, appearing first as memory decline and, over several years, destroying cognition, personality, and ability to function. Confusion and restlessness may also occur.

The type, severity, sequence, and progression of mental changes vary widely across individuals. The early symptoms of AD, which include forgetfulness and loss of concentration, can easily be missed because they resemble the natural signs of aging. Similar symptoms can also result from fatigue, grief, depression, illness, vision or hearing loss, the use of alcohol or certain medications, or simply the burden of having too many details to remember at once.

Alzheimer's is a progressive disease, and the course it follows varies from person to person. Some have the disease only for the last 5 years of life, while others may have it for as many as 20 years. The most common cause of death in AD patients is infection, which can vary in type (for instance, bacterial, chlamydeous or pneumonic.)

Again, Alzheimer's is primarily a disease of the aged. In fact, 90 percent of AD occurs in people who are over 65 years of age, and the number of new cases *doubles* in each decade of life after 65. Epidemiologists estimate that perhaps half of those persons older than 85 may have AD. About 5 million Americans and 15 million other people worldwide are believed to currently have Alzheimer's disease. And given the aging of the general population, these numbers will likely increase in the near future.

WHAT CAUSES ALZHEIMER'S DISEASE?

Different theories abound as to what causes Alzheimer's disease. The so-called *amyloid cascade hypothesis* is currently the most widely held explanation. Basically, it assumes that the beta-amyloid protein deposits are toxic to the brain, as they interrupt or interfere with the normal signaling that takes place.

Another theory is that AD results from toxicity due to heavy metals. Aluminum is a major suspect, and several research studies have found more than a casual association. Sources of aluminum include pots and pans, antacids, and so on. Exactly what happens is not known, but the theory is that the aluminum knocks out the enzymes/proteins that are important for the proper digestion of certain compounds that become toxic if allowed to build up. A bunch of these enzymes may be at play.

This process can be explained by the *lock-and-key hypothesis of enzyme functionality*. To understand this hypothesis, you need to know that an enzyme, which is usually a protein or a glycoprotein, has a certain structure. That structure has to be exactly correct for the enzyme to function correctly. More specifically, the structure has to allow the enzyme to fit onto its *substrate*, or its food. Without such a fit, the enzyme cannot work. Why?

Suppose the enzyme looks like a little Pac-Man, but the jaws don't have to move to eat things well. The jaws do need to be open, however.

Also, the shape of the mouth has to fit the identification sequence, or the area on the target (that is, the substrate), in such a way that it resembles how a key fits into a lock. Consider it a tight fit—very tight! Well, it isn't uncommon for a heavy metal to knock out an enzyme. And if the enzyme has a certain structure, the heavy metal can come in and bind to the enzyme. Where it binds is important because it may or may not initiate a change in the structure of the enzyme. When it does cause a change, it's known as a *conformational change*.

Suppose the heavy metal binds away from the mouth of the Pac-Man. (It can either bind there or actually in the active site, but let's say it binds on the opposite side.) That binding can also cause the enzyme to change its structure. If it does change, it will make the Pac-Man's mouth become twisted or disfigured in someway. Pac-Man will have a cleft lip of sorts, and because of that, the mouth will no longer be able to fit around the food it has to eat. In other words, the Pac-Man enzyme won't be able to eat the substrate.

So, what happens when enzymes are not functional (or at least, not optimally functional)? Understandably, their food—or the substrates we are interested in—will not get eaten, which is bad. That uneaten food, which is comprised of proteins or components of proteins called *peptides*, will build up in the body. The production of peptides and proteins is very tightly regulated: They are produced at a particular time, in a particular place, and all of that follows an exact schedule. That's normal. It's also normal for the enzymes to digest these peptides so that they can be removed by other body systems.

If that doesn't happen, for whatever reason, then disease can set in. When these proteins or peptides build up, they form structures known as *plaques*. These plaques are actually cytotoxic, which means they kill cells. In the case of Alzheimer's disease, the plaques build up in the brain, impairing the proper functioning of the nerve cells and killing the tissue around the sites where they decide to locate.

The brain is made up mainly of nerve cells, and like all cells, each nerve cell has a cell membrane. That membrane is composed of *phospholipids*, which are fat molecules with phosphates attached to them. All cells have phospholipids. If a cell does not have them or does not have them in the correct amounts, then the integrity of the cellular membrane will be weakened.

HOW IS ALZHEIMER'S DISEASE TREATED?

Alzheimer's disease, first described by the German physician Alois Alzheimer in 1907, has proven difficult to diagnose and treat, in part, because many of its symptoms can be associated with other conditions. For instance, the accumulation of protein as plaque outside nerve cells occurs only in people with Alzheimer's, whereas the twisting and tangling of protein fibers that usually occurs inside nerve cells may also occur in people with *other* brain diseases. Likewise, damage to the *hippocampus* region of the brain, which can interfere with memory processing and cause various blood vessel disorders and deficiencies of neurotransmitters (chemicals that allow neurons to communicate with each other), occurs in people with Alzheimer's but not exclusively so. Thus, age-related dementia can result from many factors.

Alzheimer's disease is currently diagnosed by *neuropsychological testing*, which involves administering a series of paper-and-pencil-type tests that measure specific aspects of an individual's cognitive functioning—for instance, IQ, memory, organizational ability, and so on. These are standardized tests, which means an individual's scores are compared to a large set of baseline data; doing so shows how much he or she deviates from what's considered normal. Neuropsychological tests are highly accurate, with a predictive accuracy rate of 80% to 95%.

Imaging tests—such as *positron emission tomography (PET) scans* and *computer-assisted tomography (CAT) scans*—may become more important diagnostic tools in the future. These tests are noninvasive (that is, they don't involve cutting into the body), yet they provide detailed images of the structures in a selected plane of tissue—the brain, for instance. By examining the images from a PET scan, doctors can identify areas of the brain that have been damaged. Identifying specific brain lesions can only be done after the patient's death, and interestingly, the number of lesions doesn't always correlate to the degree of dementia. Regardless, an autopsy is needed to provide the definitive diagnosis of Alzheimer's.

A CAT scan can also be used to help establish the presence of other disorders that mimic Alzheimer's disease (some of which are reversible), but it can't be used alone in the first stages of the disease to make a definitive diagnosis. In later stages, a CAT scan can often show the changes that are characteristic of AD, such as an atrophied (shrunken) brain with widened tissue indentations and enlarged cerebral ventricles (fluid-filled chambers). But again, a CAT scan isn't really useful in *diagnosing* Alzheimer's at the start.

There is no cure for Alzheimer's disease and no way to slow its progression. For some people in the early or middle stages of the disease, taking a medication such as tacrine may alleviate some cognitive symptoms. Mild to moderate dementia of the Alzheimer's type can also be treated with Aricept (donepezil) and Exelon (rivastigmine). Both of these are *reversible acetylcholinesterase (ACE) inhibitors* and help treat the loss of memory and thinking ability associated with Alzheimer's. (ACE is a neurotransmitter that's important to proper brain functioning; the more we have, the better.)

Other medications can be used to help control the behavioral symptoms of AD, such as sleeplessness, agitation, wandering, anxiety, and depression. These treatments are aimed at making the patient more comfortable.

WHAT IS THE PROBIOTIC SOLUTION?

The use of probiotics has several important implications in treating and even preventing Alzheimer's. For instance, taking phosphatidyl serine (PS) can restore the weakened cell membrane that's thought to lead to the disease. PS can be produced in the body and also introduced by ingesting things such as eggs and supplements. Doing so will ensure that every living organism in the body—the bacteria as well as the cells—will contain membranes composed mainly of phospholipids. Even if a cell is dead, the phospholipids will be in great shape (providing the cell does not die from poor phospholipid constitution).

Taking PS has both prophylactic (that is, preventive) and therapeutic purposes. Any cell that's starting along the road toward death (and remember, all cells eventually die) will be much more stable and much happier if you give it a supply of PS. With this boost, the cell will be better able to fend off the ill effects of accumulated toxins. Remember that the plaques that build up in the body kill cells. It's been shown that taking large doses of PS (for instance, 300 milligrams per day) can slow or stop the pathogenic effects of AD.

Now, if you start ingesting a bunch of bacteria, many of them will die. This is actually good because the cell wall components of these bacteria, most of which are phospholipids, will become available for absorption by the body. (We'll discuss later why we *want* some of the probiotics to be alive.) This will slow down or stop the degenerative process that characterizes AD.

Can the degenerative process that characterizes Alzheimer's be reversed? To some degree, yes. Supplementing with PS and the like can bring improvement because it helps the body deal with the peptides. Even so, in AD, it seems that the body just can't keep pace with the amount of peptides being produced. This may be because an enzyme has been knocked out or attenuated (that is, made to function suboptimally). If the *production* of peptides could be slowed down, it might be possible for body to process them on its own and thus remove the offending particles.

As an aside, there may be natural ingredients that can increase the body's production of those enzymes responsible for removing peptides. It may even be that components of bacteria can do this. In fact, it's well known that the body can absorb intact enzymes from the gastrointestinal tract. It's also well known that probiotics produce a large variety of enzymes and usually at very high levels. (We will discuss this in more detail in Chapter 5 on lactose intolerance.) Given all this, it's not only conceivable but probable that taking large doses of probiotics and having their enzymes absorbed into circulation will cause many of the offending particles to be digested before they have an opportunity to accumulate and produce plaques in the brain. Again, it's the accumulation of these plaques over time that's thought to be responsible for AD.

Mitochondrial dysfunction is also thought to be at play here. The mitochondria are the powerhouses of the cell, supplying it with energy. When the mitochondria don't function properly, there's an increase in the accumulation of free radicals and also fluxes in the calcium level. Both of these effects are significant in terms of AD.

A *free radical* is a molecule that has an uneven number of electrons; as such, it has an open (or half) bond and is highly reactive. The production of free radicals is a normal part of the body's living process; in fact, they are produced all the time. But usually, mechanisms are in place to control free radicals and eliminate them once produced. When free radicals are allowed to accumulate, they go after healthy cells. They are like little lightning, zapping other cells and producing even more free radicals.

Having too much calcium in the body is also harmful. Why? Calcium is intimately involved in a process called *signal transduction*. Basically, this involves taking a signal from outside a cell to inside and affecting the DNA. When this happens to nerve cells, it affects the voltage gradient required for the passage of electrical impulses. Calcium is a charged molecule, and changing the amount of calcium inside or outside a cell can change the level of current that cell is able to generate.

Probiotics can help stabilize the level of calcium. If a large amount of calcium is ingested, for instance, then the probiotics will be able to consume much of it. And what the probiotics don't consume, they will push out of the body along with the normal waste material. Also, calcium is usually bound, so if there is too little, the probiotics will help liberate the calcium from a bound state.

Isoflavones (naturally occurring, weakly estrogenic compounds that are usually derived from soy) have also been shown to be important for AD in a sort of round-about way. There is a protein called *tau* that's regulated by estrogen and estrogen-like compounds, such as the isoflavones found in plants and, in particular, in soy. There are two types of isoflavones: those with and without a sugar (*glycone* and *aglycone*, respectively). Isoflavones are big and bulky when the sugar is attached; in order for them to be absorbed, the sugar has to be removed. This is done by an enzyme called *glucosidase* (literally, "sugar cleaver"), which cuts the sugar from the isoflavone molecule and allows for absorption. This *must* happen before the body can use the isoflavone.

Products such as Fermasoy have been fermented with probiotics to create a protein powder that's high in aglycone isoflavone—the sugar-carrying type. Consuming these products not only provides a high-quality protein but also a relatively high level of the absorbable isoflavone.

Not all probiotics can create the sugarless isoflavones at the same level. Certain ones have been tested and selected for their various abilities. The MAKTech process of strain validation and certification is designed to optimize just this sort of parameter. (For contact information, see the Resources section at the end of the book.) This will be discussed in more detail in Chapter 10 on probiotic delivery systems, but basically, DNA fingerprinting and various other molecular biology and biochemical analyses are performed to identify the optimal strains and ingredients for a particular use.

Given that the "baby boom" generation is fast approaching the age at which early onset AD is detected, it's vital that we learn more about this disease. Doing so is of particular importance when we consider that many of the people who run our governments are at or near this age. The Alzheimer's diagnosis of former President Ronald Reagan shortly after he left office was shocking to many Americans, given the potential implications of his condition.

Until a cure for AD is found, taking probiotics may serve a valuable purpose in at least slowing the progression of the disease. And in terms of improving the quality of life for people with AD, as well as those around them, this would have an enormous and far-reaching impact.

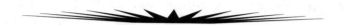

CHAPTER 5

How Probiotics Can Help Counteract the Effects of Lactose Intolerance

WHAT IS LACTOSE INTOLERANCE?

Lactose intolerance is the inability to digest significant amounts of *lactose*, the predominant sugar found in milk. This inability results from a shortage of the enzyme *lactase*, which is normally produced by the cells that line the small intestine. Lactase breaks down milk sugar into simpler forms that can then be absorbed into the bloodstream.

What happens when there is not enough lactase to digest the amount of lactose consumed? The results may be very distressing, although not usually dangerous. Common symptoms include nausea, cramps, bloating, gas, and diarrhea, which begin about 30 minutes to 2 hours after eating or drinking foods containing lactose.

The severity of the symptoms varies, depending on the amount of lactose the individual can tolerate. Most people, even those diagnosed as lactose intolerant, can consume one glass of milk—which contains between 10 and 12 grams of lactose—without experiencing symptoms. Others, of course, will have problems with less than that amount. Finally, not everyone who is deficient in lactase has symptoms; only those who do are considered lactose intolerant.

Between 30 and 50 million Americans are lactose intolerant, and the condition is more prevalent in certain ethnic and racial populations. As many as 75 percent of all African Americans and American Indians and 90 percent of Asian Americans are lactose intolerant. The condition is least common among persons of Northern European descent.

Lactose intolerance is also age related, as the incidence of this condition increases with age. Among older adults (that is, over age 50), approximately 46 percent have problems with lactose intolerance, compared with only 26 percent of young adults (under 50). And among those in the 60 to 69 age bracket, 65 percent report symptoms of lactose intolerance, with 3 percent reporting symptoms as "severe."

WHAT CAUSES LACTOSE INTOLERANCE?

Some of the causes of lactose intolerance are well known. For instance, certain digestive diseases and injuries to the small intestine can reduce the amount of enzymes produced. In rare cases, children are born without the ability to produce lactase, the enzyme that digests lactose; this is called *congenital-type lactose intolerance*. But for most people, lactase deficiency is a condition that develops naturally over time. After about the age of 2, the body begins to produce less lactase, and that level continues to drop off through adolescence and into old age. Thus, many people may not experience symptoms until they are much older; this is called *adult-type lactose intolerance*.

Before going any further with this discussion, let's clarify the meanings of a few terms. As noted earlier, *lactose* is a sugar. Strictly speaking, it's a complex sugar, meaning that it contains more than one type. Lactose contains two sugars, so it's often referred to as a *disaccharide*. (The di- is for "two," and the *saccharide* is for "sugar.") Lactose has one glucose and one galactose stuck together. These are very similar sugars and differ only in their arrangement of certain bonds.

The human body normally can produce enzymes that digest

disaccharides. Each different disaccharide requires its own enzyme for production and for digestion. Again, lactose is digested by an enzyme called *lactase*, which is also more precisely known as *beta-galactosidase*, or simply *beta-gal*. (This enzyme is sold over the counter in a purified form to treat lactose intolerance.) When ingested, beta-gal separates the glucose and the galactose elements of the lactose, freeing them up so they can be used by the body to create other things. For instance, the bacterial flora can use both as food, so they are readily consumed.

Remember that *lactase* and *beta-gal* are the same enzyme and have the same function: to digest *lactose*. And when the body has too little of this enzyme, the result is *lactose intolerance*.

Diagnosis of Lactose Intolerance

The most common tests used to measure the absorption of lactose in the digestive system are the lactose tolerance test, the hydrogen breath test, and the stool acidity test. Each of these tests is performed on an outpatient basis at a hospital, clinic, or doctor's office.

The *lactose tolerance test* begins with the individual fasting for a set period of time and then drinking a liquid that contains lactose. After that, several blood samples are taken over a two-hour period to measure the person's blood glucose (or blood sugar) level, which indicates how well the body is able to digest lactose. Normally, when lactose reaches the digestive system, it's broken down into glucose and galactose by the enzyme lactase. The liver then changes the galactose into glucose, which enters the bloodstream and raises the blood glucose level. If the lactose is not completely broken down, the blood glucose level will not rise, confirming a diagnosis of lactose intolerance.

The second test, the *hydrogen breath test*, measures the amount of hydrogen in the patient's breath. Normally, there is very little, but when undigested lactose in the colon is fermented by bacteria, various gases are produced, including hydrogen. The hydrogen is absorbed from the intestines, carried through the bloodstream to the lungs, and exhaled. In this test, the patient drinks a lactose-loaded beverage, and the breath is analyzed at regular intervals. A raised level of hydrogen in his or her breath will indicate the improper digestion of lactose. Certain foods, medications, and cigarettes can affect the accuracy of this test and should be avoided before taking it.

The lactose tolerance and hydrogen breath tests should not be given to infants and very young children who are suspected of having lactose intolerance. The lactose loading involved in both these tests may be dangerous for very young individuals because they are more prone to dehydration, which can result from having diarrhea in reaction to the lactose. When a baby or young child has symptoms of lactose intolerance, many pediatricians recommend changing from cow's milk to soy formula and waiting for the symptoms to go away.

If necessary, infants and young children may be diagnosed using a *stool acidity test*, which measures the amount of acid in the stool. Undigested lactose that has been fermented by bacteria in the colon will create lactic acid and other short-chain fatty acids that can be detected. In addition, glucose may be present in the sample as a result of unabsorbed lactose in the colon.

HOW IS LACTOSE INTOLERANCE TREATED?

As mentioned earlier, congenital lactase deficiency is extremely rare. Suffice it to say that this type of condition can be treated using the measures recommended in this section. Again, however, treatment should be scaled back for infants and young children, as they are prone to the dehydration that can result from having diarrhea. Many pediatricians simply recommend giving the young children soy formula instead of cow's milk and waiting for symptoms to abate.

Avoiding milk and dairy products would seem the obvious solution to lactose intolerance; however, drinking milk can have very beneficial health effects. Milk and dairy products, in general, contain many things that are good for the human body. In addition to the sugars already discussed, they contain high levels of proteins, substances that control hormones (such as glyco-macro peptide), and antiviral compounds (such as 3'-sialyl lactose, or 3').

When people notice that they cannot digest straight milk or dairy, they tend to ingest fermented products, which are tolerable. Yogurt is one of the most popular fermented dairy products. It contains a high level of beta-gal, which does a number of things. Specifically, the beta-gal can delay the time it takes food to pass through the gastrointestinal (GI) tract, and it has positive effects on intestinal function and colonic bacterial flora (that is, friendly bacteria). Most notably, it reduces the symptoms of lactose intolerance.

Although milk and foods made from milk are the only natural sources of lactose, it can be found in many other foods. In fact, lactose is often added to prepared foods because it's so cheap. Lactose is often used as a filler to make a product meet a designated weight or shape. For instance, suppose a single vitamin capsule is supposed to weigh 500 milligrams, but after all of the ingredients have been added together, it weighs only 450 milligrams. By law, the manufacturer has to make that capsule weigh 500 milligrams. Of course, they want to correct this problem as cheaply as possible, and so they add 50 milligrams of lactose. The same thing is done with certain food products, too.

Unfortunately, product-labeling laws allow lactose to be included at levels that don't have to be reported. This means that you could eat lactose in something and not even know it, which is an obvious problem if you have very low tolerance. Thus, it's important to know about the many food products that may contain lactose, even in small amounts, including these:

- bread and other baked goods
- processed breakfast cereals
- instant potatoes, soups, and breakfast drinks
- margarine
- lunch meats (other than kosher)
- salad dressings
- candies and other snacks
- mixes for pancakes, biscuits, and cookies

Some products labeled "nondairy," such as powdered coffee creamers and whipped toppings, may also include ingredients that are derived from milk and therefore contain lactose.

As noted, lactose is a common filler for a number of pharmaceuticals and over-the-counter drugs. It's used as the base for more than 20 percent of prescription drugs and about 6 percent of over-the-counter medicines. Many types of birth control pills, for example, contain lactose, as do some tablets for treating stomach acid and gas. However, these products typically affect only people with severe lactose intolerance.

If you or a family member is lactose intolerant, be a smart shopper and learn to read food labels with care. Look not only for milk and lactose among the contents on product labels but also such words as *whey, curds, milk by-products, dry milk solids*, and *nonfat dry milk powder*. If any of these is listed on the label, the product contains lactose.

WHAT IS THE PROBIOTIC SOLUTION?

Normally, when lactose is ingested, the body finds a way to digest it. The body will either take the lactose and use its own beta-gal enzyme (that is, lactase) to cut the lactose into its constituent parts (that is, glucose and galactose), which get absorbed and utilized by the body, or the body will use the lactase from the resident probiotics in the gut. When the body is lactose intolerant, however, the lactose is not broken down by beta-gal, for whatever reason. When that happens, the lactose rapidly passes through the GI tract and enters into the colon.

For the sake of argument, suppose that the level of beta-gal is low because the level of probiotics (which contain very high levels of this enzyme) is low due to some disease state or other condition. As mentioned elsewhere in this book, having low numbers of probiotic (or good) organisms is associated with having high numbers of pathogenic (or bad) organisms. Having a few pathogenic organisms in the GI tract is normal because they will be kept in check by a variety of factors.

(Besides, it would be impossible to eliminate all of the bad bacteria.) Having a lot of bad bacteria is a problem, however, because both the probiotics and the pathogenic bacteria can feed on lactose. (You may be wondering if lactose is a prebiotic, and the answer is no. The reason is that by definition, a *prebiotic* has to stimulate the *probiotics*, not the pathogenic organisms. Here, both can feed on lactose.)

If there is a low number of probiotics and a high number of pathogenics, guess what is feeding on the lactose? Right! The pathogenic bacteria. This is bad for all the obvious reasons plus one more: Pathogenic organisms form gas. In fact, they are sometimes referred to as *gas-formers*. Probiotics, on the other hand, form very little, if any, gas under normal conditions. Gas causes *distention*, or swelling of the intestines, which is painful (as anyone who has tried to hold it back for any length of time already knows). And having gas leads to flatulence (or passing gas), which has its own unpleasant effects.

Diarrhea is another major problem for the person who is lactose intolerant. Normally, lactose does not get into the colon intact; it's digested before it arrives there. But with lactose intolerance, the lactose passes through the GI tract quickly and into the colon (which is part of the large intestine). This is where the water involved in digestion is usually absorbed. If there is a high level of lactose in the colon, the water will not be absorbed. This is what causes diarrhea.

These symptoms of lactose intolerance can be treated using products on the market that contain purified beta-gal (or lactase). There are also so-called lactose-free products; for the most part, the lactase enzyme has been added to these products, and by the time you ingest them, all the lactose has been munched up.

A folk remedy for treating lactose intolerance is to eat fresh yogurt, which can contain a level of probiotics that is in the 100s of billions per milliliter. This is one of the reasons we know that consuming very high levels of probiotics is safe. For years, people have been ingesting far higher levels of probiotics in foods such as yogurt than are currently found in most capsule-type supplements. To avoid having symptoms of maldigestion, it appears that at least 10 to 20 billion organisms are required per episode of lactose exposure. In this case, if a little is good, more is better.

So, you can either add probiotics to your system by eating yogurt or by consuming them in capsule form using one of the delivery systems mentioned in Chapter 10. Again, the rule is to use a high level of probiotics, and generally, the more varied, the better. However, each body is different, so it's best to try different strains. Maintaining the high level of each strain of probiotics is important because each strain has unique features that it will bring to the metabolic activities of the intestines. And depending on what probiotics are already in the GI tract, the strains can have different survival rates. Some are more resistant than others to the gastric environment and bile. And in this case, you *don't* want the most resistant ones.

The probiotic organisms that are very resistant are usually touted as such; in fact, that quality is used as a selling point, promising that you will get implantation, which many companies say is crucial to functionality. This is just wrong in some cases—and with lactose intolerance, in particular. But why?

When you have lactose intolerance, the situation is acute and immediate. You need to digest the enzymes in the probiotics *quickly* so they will come into contact with the lactose already in your system. Otherwise, the lactose will move rapidly through your GI tract, wreaking havoc. The way to ensure that quick contact is to deliver the enzyme (that is, beta-gal or lactase) at a high level. So, be aware that different probiotics produce different levels of enzymes.

Now, when probiotics are added to the body, the enzymes they contain are basically encapsulated, or physically separated from the lactose. Think of probiotics as "bags" of enzymes. When the bags hit the stomach, some will actually break open and some won't, depending on the hardiness of the strain. For instance, *Lactobacillus rhamnosus* and *Lactobacillus acidophilus* are very resistant. They can pass through the stomach and into the GI intact, rather than deliver the beta-gal into the small intestine.

Compare what happens with strains like *Streptococcus thermophilus* and *Lactobacillus bulgaricus*, both of which are much less resistant to the hostile gastric environment. They will largely have been broken down before they reach the GI, so their beta-gal enzymes will be released into the GI tract. The beta-gal will then be free to contact the lactose and digest it properly. So, what you should really look for is a high-dose, multistrain probiotic product. That way, both the gastric and the intestinal environments will be covered.

Some manufacturers will try to misinform you to get you to buy their products, saying that a certain portion of the probiotics that release their enzymes due to low resistance to the gastric juices will have their enzymes digested. It's true—some of them will. The operative word is *some*. That's why it's important to supplement with such large numbers of organisms. This is, after all, a game of numbers.

That principle underlies the *Brudnak method* of pulsing and rotating probiotics during supplementation. Here's how you can make it work for you: If you ingest a lot of lactose in a meal, pulse by taking high levels of probiotics at the same time. I prefer to use a product that has a mixed culture, since some will be destroyed and some will be delivered intact into the intestines. But mainly, you want nonresistant, wimpy-type probiotics.

This brings up the question of when to take probiotics: before a meal, during a meal, or after a meal? There has been a lot of debate about this (some of it, rather silly), so I will try to explain it in a very straightforward manner. First, it depends on *why* you are taking the probiotics. If you are taking them as a general supplement and have no immediate concerns, then take them with a meal. The food will not only raise the pH of the stomach but also provide a degree of physical protection for the probiotics. If, however, you are taking the probiotics to treat a condition like lactose intolerance, then you should take them just before a meal so as to take advantage of the gastric juices in liberating the enzymes. Don't take the probiotics too long before a meal because you don't want all the enzymes to be destroyed by the hydrochloric acid in your stomach.

There is also a lot of discussion about whether probiotics can be taken with enzyme supplements. Let's think about that. We have discussed the use of enzymes that are naturally present in probiotics. In addition to lactase, probiotics contain lipases, proteases and peptidases, and many more enzymes. We know that probiotics are constantly breaking open and releasing their enzymes, which come in contact with other probiotics and human tissues. We also know that this causes no problems and, in fact, is often a good thing. And we know that probiotics and enzymes are naturally present in fermented foods and all eaten together.

Some people argue that certain enzymes can digest the attachment sites for probiotics and thus should not be taken with together. While that may occur *on occasion*, for the most part, those attachment sites are hard to get to and designed such that only probiotics can "see" them. In fact, the attachment sites are usually shielded by a very protective covering called a *glycocalix*, which is designed to prevent this very sort of digestion from occurring. Also, the probiotics themselves have evolved an outer layer that's resistant to enzymatic degradation. Yes, some small amount will be digested, but it's nothing to worry about.

In sum, your probiotics and enzymes will function perfectly well when taken together. If you hear a manufacturer trying to suggest otherwise, I recommend buying another product! In my opinion, common sense and knowledge of biological systems both dictate that response. Look into Matol Botanical International, which has a great product that combines enzymes and probiotics because they do work so well together. (For contact information, see the Resources section at the end of the book.)

Supplementing with probiotics is worth investigating if you have lactose intolerance. I've been doing it for years and have been very happy with the results. I also recommend supplementation to my clients when appropriate, with the same good results, and if you have problems with lactose intolerance, I suggest you try taking probiotics, as well.

It will be exciting to see the outcomes of research in this area in the near future and beyond. Given our aging population, the fact that lactose intolerance is more common among the elderly means that we can expect more research about and more products for treating this condition.

The Probiotics Potential for Preventing Diabetes and for Effective Weight Control

WHAT IS DIABETES?

Diabetes is a group of metabolic disorders that result in hyperglycemia due to decreased insulin production or inefficient insulin utilization. Put simply, there is too much sugar in the blood and the body does not use it correctly.

There are two types of diabetes. In *type I diabetes* (also called *insulin-dependent diabetes mellitus*), the body produces little or no insulin; this is considered an autoimmune disease. Because this type of diabetes is often diagnosed early in life, it's sometimes referred to as *juvenile-onset diabetes*. In *type II diabetes* (or *noninsulin-dependent diabetes mellitus*), the body has a reduced ability to control blood sugar. Because this type of diabetes is often diagnosed later in life, it's sometimes called *adult-onset diabetes*.

Diabetes is a very significant health problem in terms of scope. Worldwide, it's the single most common metabolic disorder. An estimated 6 percent of the American population is diabetic, or around 16 million people. Most of these people have type II diabetes, making it a major cause of heart disease, kidney disease, stroke, blindness, and early death.

Weight control, a related issue, is also a significant worldwide problem, particularly in the United States and other Western developed countries. It's generally agreed that the tendency among Westerners to be overweight is due to a sedentary lifestyle and high-fat diet. In a recent U.S. poll, 65 percent of the respondents described themselves as being from 5 to more than 30 pounds overweight. A study by the National Health and Nutrition Examination had the same results, finding that the percentage of overweight American adults is now at 64.5 percent. And sadly, this trend holds true for children, too, who are becoming obese at an alarming rate.

Two disturbing conclusions can be drawn from studies such as these. First, the findings cut across age, gender, and race, which means people are overweight throughout American society, not just among certain groups. And second, the percentage of the population that is overweight has increased steadily since the 1970s.

WHAT CAUSES DIABETES?

In most cases, diabetes is believed to be caused by a genetic disorder, in which the pancreas fails to produce and secrete enough insulin. But for type II diabetes, certain lifestyle factors are strongly associated not only with its onset but also with the ability to treat it effectively. Central among those factors is being overweight. People who are overweight are twice as likely to develop type II diabetes as those who are not overweight.

The relationship between being overweight and developing diabetes is a kind of "chicken or egg" thing. In fact, the relationship between obesity and insulin resistance is extremely complex. Scientists are only beginning to make headway in their understanding of it. What is known, however, is that as someone becomes obese, his or her body tends to lose its sensitivity to insulin.

Insulin is known as the "fat hormone" because it helps the body utilize glucose and make fat when there is extra energy around in the form of food. Quite simply, insulin works like this: It's secreted by special cells of the pancreas and functions by binding to receptors on the surfaces of cells. And through a complex signaling mechanism, the insulin tells the cells to use the glucose.

In addition to insulin, certain circulating hormones also play a role in diabetes and weight control. For instance, the hormone *leptin* controls, to a large extent, the body's ability to respond to insulin and also induces feelings of satiety in the brain. Think of it as the "I'm full" hormone because it tells your body that you have had enough to eat.

Having diabetes can also lead to a host of health problems, including retinal degeneration, blindness, and kidney and nerve damage. Diabetes can be a contributing cause of atherosclerosis, which is the most common type of arteriosclerosis (hardening and thickening of the arteries). In extreme cases, the poor circulation that results from this condition can lead to amputation and even death.

Being overweight also increases the risks for other health problems, such as heart disease and stroke, certain types of cancer, gout (joint pain caused by excess uric acid), and gall bladder disease. Being overweight can also cause problems such as sleep apnea (interrupted breathing during sleep) and osteoarthritis (wearing away of the joints). And the more overweight you are, the more likely you are to have health problems.

HOW IS DIABETES TREATED?

For someone with type II diabetes, losing weight and becoming more physically active can help control his or her blood sugar level. For someone who uses medicine (that is, insulin) to help control his or her blood sugar, making these lifestyle changes may make it possible to decrease the amount of medication needed. What we are mostly concerned with is type II, as dietary intervention is a primary factor in making a healthy lifestyle change. But even with a major dietary modification, type II diabetes requires monitoring the blood glucose level at least daily and often before and after each meal.

Weight loss can also help improve the harmful effects that come from being overweight. For someone who is overweight, losing as little as 5 percent to 10 percent of his or her body weight may improve many of these effects, such as having high blood pressure and developing diabetes. Even a small weight loss can improve someone's health.

However, many overweight people have difficulty reaching their healthy body weight. Making long-term changes in eating and physical activity habits is the best way to lose weight and keep it off over time. To be safe, weight loss should be slow and steady—no more than 1 pound per week. Very rapid weight loss can cause the loss of muscle, rather than fat, and also increases the chances of developing other problems, such as gallstones, gout, and nutrient deficiencies.

If you are not overweight but know that health problems related to being overweight run in your family, you should try to keep your weight steady and at a healthy level. And if you have family members with weight-related health problems, you are more likely to develop them yourself. If you are not sure of your risk of developing weight-related health problems, including diabetes, you should talk to your health care provider.

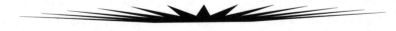

What Is the Probiotic Solution?

In this discussion of diabetes and its relationship to probiotics, the issue of weight control will be in the background. In other words, you should always bear in mind that *diabetes and weight control are directly related*. Also, what's said about type II diabetes can loosely be applied to type I diabetes, as well, at least in so far as the use of probiotics goes.

Three basic strategies are used to treat diabetes: (1) to reduce glucose absorption from the intestines by either dietary restrictions or drugs; (2) to reduce glucose synthesis in the liver; and (3) to increase the metabolic utilization of glucose. Probiotics can play a key role in the first and the third strategies but have only a minimal effect in the second strategy, so we won't cover it in this discussion. Given all this, taking probiotics is probably not the complete answer for treating diabetes and assisting with weight control, but it can serve an important function.

The first treatment strategy—to reduce glucose absorption in the gastrointestinal (GI) tract—can be assisted by a variety of good products that block sugar absorption. One such product is Sweetease, which is produced by AdvoCare. (For contact information about this and other manufacturers, see the Resources section at the end of the book.) Another very similar product is MAKSwee-T (pronounced "mak-swee-TEA"), which contains the proprietarily processed and naturally occurring *L. arabinose*. MAKSwee-T is a really interesting substance in that it is not digested to any great extent by humans but is digested by probiotics, such as *Lactobacillus plantarum*. As such, MAKSwee-T would make a wonderful *prebiotic* in a combination prebiotic/probiotic product. It also inhibits gastrointestinal sucrase, so the body doesn't make fat using the ordinary table sugar found in most diets. Not only that, but it tastes good—really sweet! I don't believe it can be sold as a sweetener, so it's labeled a "flavor enhancer" or a "prebiotic."

In this treatment strategy, the goal is to use a very high dose of probiotics in order to prevent the food from being digested by the body and turned into fat. Put differently, the food that would ordinarily be absorbed will be consumed by the probiotics. So, you can have your cake and the probiotics will eat it, too! One particularly interesting product that's been developed with this principle in mind is called PerfectContours by HLN. It contains very high levels of *Lactobacillus acidophilus, Lactobacillus rhamnosus, Bifidobacterium bifidum,* and the MAKSwee-T enzyme inhibitor (to block sugar absorption and utilization for the production of fat). This sort of formula represents the next generation in products for people with diabetes and for those who want to maintain a normal weight. Moreover, it is ephedra free and body friendly.

Glucose can actually present itself in the intestines in many different forms. As noted earlier, glucose can be associated with other sugars to form more complex ones, which are then broken down by the body to liberate the glucose, allowing it to be absorbed. For instance, in order for the body to break down sucrose into its basic components (fructose and glucose) and then absorb these sugars, there must be sucrase in the intestines. Probiotics can play a role here because just like pathogenic bacteria, they will feed on glucose. Actually, *everything* in the body loves glucose! It's a basic energy source and easy for all organisms to use. The metabolic machinery of nearly every organism uses glucose as its primary energy source.

Given this, what can be done in the intestines to help treat diabetes and assist in weight control? Let's take a situation in which you eat a bunch of sugar. (To keep things simple, the sugar will be glucose, but what's said will essentially hold true for other sugars, as well.) If you eat pure glucose, what will happen? Assuming you don't go into a diabetic coma, much of the glucose will be absorbed initially. To do that, it has to pass into the intestines and get by whatever is surrounding the intestinal epithelial cells, if anything. In a healthy gut, probiotics are surrounding those cells (or layered on top of them, as I like to visualize it), and in an unhealthy gut, there are a bunch more pathogenic bacteria.

Regardless, the glucose is then absorbed into the intestinal epithelial cells, and from there, it gets passed on to other parts of the body. (Of course, this is assuming that not all of the glucose gets used there. Most of it won't, as the epithelial cells tend to like other sources of energy just as well and are designed to pass on glucose.) In sum, the probiotics lining the GI tract provide a first line of defense against high-level glucose absorption. That means that if you were to supplement with huge amounts of probiotics, you would greatly strengthen that line of defense because probiotics preferentially utilize glucose.

So, is glucose a *prebiotic*? No! By definition, a prebiotic has to selectively feed the probiotics and not the pathogenic organisms, such as yeast, *E. coli*, and the like. That still doesn't change the fact that the probiotics really want the glucose. They won't even touch other sugars to any large extent if glucose is around in large quantities. The reason for this preference is simple: Feeding on glucose requires very little effort by the probiotics. All life conforms to this cost/benefit ratio. The easier something is to do, the greater the chance that the life will do it, provided it brings some benefit. Probiotics have mechanisms in place to use the glucose, so they will bring it in and happily munch away on it.

Now, back to our sugar-eating example: If you have a whole bunch of probiotics in there, all voraciously consuming glucose, then there will be less glucose available for transport throughout the body. The net result will be a lower amount of glucose in the blood. And if there is lower blood glucose, there will be less glucose available to the liver for the creation of glycogen (and all the other things it does), which is the body's way of storing glucose. Finally, if less glycogen is created, then over time, there will be less stored glycogen available for the body to make glucose when it needs it. And remember, this all happens simply by supplying large amounts of probiotics.

If consuming large of numbers of probiotics is so beneficial, why not really boost the process by consuming some of the other organisms found naturally in the intestines, such as yeast and *E. coli?* The danger in doing that may seem obvious, but let me explain why, nonetheless, as some people have made that extension and do use these potentially dangerous organisms.

By supplementing your diet with large numbers of *E. coli* or yeast, you are just asking for an infection. Yes, doing so will absolutely have an effect (and even stimulate the heck out of your immune system), but again, consider the cost/benefit ratio. Death is far too high a cost for the limited benefit that might be accrued by ingesting potentially dangerous organisms. Besides, if all the benefits can be achieved with probiotics, why take such an insane risk?

This brings us to the topic of weight control and its relationship to developing diabetes. Glucose is a very good energy source and readily lends itself to the production of other substances in the body. If your body has much more energy (in the form of glucose) than it can use, what will it do? It will store the glucose as extra pounds, which you may end up carrying around for the rest of your life. The formula is simple: Too much energy (that is, glucose) equals weight gain. If you take in more calories than you use, you will gain weight.

There is one exception: If you decrease the amount of glucose that passes into your body, then you will effectively decrease the amount available for weight gain. This is a very important point. Glucose and other energy sources do not contribute to your gaining weight *until they actually get into your body.* That is to say, the energy source must pass through your stomach and intestines before it can be used. It's not the act of ingesting the energy source that adds the pounds. That means that the calories you are counting are only *potential* calories until they are actually used to do something.

Here's an example: If you eat a piece of steak, that steak needs to be converted by your body into things it can use (that is, digested), and that process can only happen inside your body. If you ate some steak but didn't digest it, then those calories wouldn't count; they would only be potential calories. This is the principle behind the eating disorder known as *bulimia*, in which someone eats but then throws up the food or uses laxatives to keep the body from absorbing the food. The bulimic relies on the fact that the calories eaten are only potential calories until they are used.

As mentioned at the start of this section, there are three major strategies for treating diabetes, the third of which is to accelerate the metabolism of glucose. Without going into great detail, there are limited options as to what you can do to make the cells inside your body use more glucose. Even taking probiotics will have a limited effect, if any, on those internal workings. But you can greatly affect what goes on inside your *intestines.* In fact, what happens in there is probably much more important than what happens inside the body in general.

For this to make sense, think of the insides of your intestines as being *external* to your body. That's what scientists do! They consider the intestines to be a hollow "tube" that runs from the mouth to the anus and around which the body is wrapped. The "tube" is a useful metaphor because nothing that passes through the intestines comes into direct contact with the interior of the body. In other words, whatever you ingest enters the tube at one end and exits it at the other—but it stays in the tube the whole time. This is true not only of food but also of probiotics. They work very well in the self-contained environment of the intestines.

As mentioned before, there are more *bacteria* in the human body than there are cells. That means that probiotics, which are good bacteria, can play a major role in the overall metabolic activities of the body. This is particularly significant in the area of weight control. If you supplement your diet with even larger numbers of probiotics, you can completely overshadow your body's own ability to utilize these compounds. Very little of the food you ingest will actually be absorbed.

So, you don't believe me? Try it yourself. If you take several 100 billion organisms (that is, 5 to 10 capsules of a 20 to 40 billion probiotics per capsule product), you will notice that you get very hungry. The probiotics will be consuming the bulk of your calories, so your body will be starved. You will have the hunger issue to deal with, but if you are trying to lose weight, you will have that no matter what you do. Some products use a material such as D-limonene, a natural anorexic, in conjunction with probiotics to help reduce feelings of hunger. This doesn't mean these products cause anorexia; rather, that is just the scientific way of saying they kill the appetite.

Finding ways to control the appetite is one of many valuable applications of probiotics in the area of diabetes and weight control. This is especially significant when you consider that nearly two-thirds of Americans are overweight and that diabetes is the most common metabolic disorder in the world. Obesity and diabetes affect us all, whether we actually have one or both conditions or are simply paying to treat them in others through rising medical and insurance costs. The long-term significance of chronic obesity, by itself, cannot be underestimated in terms of its effects on society.

CHAPTER 7

Curing Yeast Infections with Probiotics

WHAT ARE YEAST INFECTIONS?

Yeast infections are caused by any of several *fungi* (plural for *fungus*) that often exist naturally in the human body. The problem occurs when there is too much of a given fungus. In effect, the bad bacteria take over and push out the good bacteria. This changes the environment (or ecology) of the body, resulting in an infection at the site of the invasion.

Yeast infections can occur in many parts of the body and in both men and women. Teenage girls and women ages 16 to 35 are most prone to vaginal yeast infections, but they can occur in girls as young as 10 or 11 and also in older women. A woman does not have to be sexually active to get a yeast infection.

One of the most common causes of yeast infections is the fungus *Candida*. Actually, there are four different types of *Candida* that can cause these infections, but nearly 80 percent are caused by a variety called *Candida albicans*. This is the variety that produces the vaginal-type yeast infections experienced by many women. *Vaginitis*, which is an inflammation of the vagina, is often caused by such an infection, as well.

Other types of yeast infections (again, commonly and collectively called *vaginitis*) are bacterial vaginosis, in which there is an overgrowth of bacteria, and yeast vaginosis, in which there is an overgrowth of yeast. Both fall into the category of urogenital tract infections, because they affect the *urogenital system (UGS)*: that is, the vagina, bladder, urethra, and so on.

The major symptom of a vaginal yeast infection is intense itching "down there." Other symptoms include vaginal discharge of a substance that is white, curdy, and mostly odorless along with soreness or rash on the outer lips of the vagina and burning, especially during urination. Not all women experience all these symptoms, but in general, if intense itching is not present, the problem is not likely a yeast infection. Some women may have discharge between menstrual periods, but this does not usually indicate a yeast infection, especially if there is no itching.

Even though itchiness is the main symptom of a yeast infection, if you have never had one before, you will find it difficult to know just what's causing your discomfort. A doctor's diagnosis will likely be needed. After that, if you should have a similar set of symptoms again, you will be better able to identify the problem or at least distinguish a yeast infection from some other condition.

Some women are more prone than others to yeast infections, for reasons that aren't entirely understood. However, it's widely believed that what causes this condition has an immunological component. This will make a great deal of sense when, later in the chapter, we discuss the use of probiotics in treating yeast infections.

WHAT CAUSES YEAST INFECTIONS?

The biggest cause of *Candida*-type yeast infections is lowered immunity, which can result from getting run down and not having enough rest or from being sick. Repeated yeast infections can be caused by certain illnesses, such as diabetes, and by physical and mental stress. Other causes include the use of antibiotics and some other medications (including birth control pills) as well as poor nutrition and significant changes in diet. In some rare cases, having repeated yeast infections may be the first sign that a woman is infected with HIV, the virus that causes AIDS. This is especially likely when yeast infections don't clear up with proper treatment. (We'll return to this subject in the next section on treatment.)

Some women get a mild yeast infection toward the end of the menstrual period, possibly in response to the body's hormonal and pH changes. These mild infections sometimes go away without treatment as the menstrual cycle progresses. Pregnant women are also more prone to developing yeast infections.

Weather conditions can also affect the likelihood of having a yeast infection. Hot, humid weather can make it easier for a yeast infection to develop. And in the winter months, wearing many layers of clothing and getting too warm indoors can increase the likelihood of infection.

Yeast infections can also be spread through sexual intercourse. A man is less likely than a woman to be aware of having a yeast infection because he may not have any symptoms. When symptoms do occur in men, they may include a moist, white, scaling rash on the penis along with itchiness or redness under the foreskin. (Even so, lowered immunity, *not* sexual transmission, is the most frequent cause of genital yeast infections in males, as it is in females.)

The best way to avoid transmitting a yeast infection through sex is to not have sex. Otherwise, using a latex condom will provide the best protection against transmission of yeast infections along with more commonly sexually transmitted diseases, including HIV infection. Individuals who are not in a committed and exclusive sexual relationship should always use a latex condom when they have sex, even if they are also using another form of birth control. And if one partner is diagnosed as having a yeast infection, both partners should be treated for it.

HOW ARE YEAST INFECTIONS TREATED?

The Food and Drug Administration (FDA) now allows medicines that were previously available only with a prescription to be sold over the counter for the treatment of recurring vaginal yeast infections. But if you've never been treated for a yeast infection, you should see your doctor before you run out and buy one of these medications. He or she may advise you to use one of these over-the-counter products or prescribe a drug called Diflucan (fluconazole). The FDA recently approved use of this drug—a tablet taken by mouth—for clearing up yeast infections with just one dose.

Over-the-counter products for vaginal yeast infections have one of four active ingredients (generic names are given first): (1) butoconazole nitrate (Femstat 3); (2) clotrimazole (Gyne-Lotrimin and others); (3) miconazole (Monistat 7 and others); and (4) tioconazole (Vagistat). These drugs all belong to the same antifungal family and work in similar ways to break down the cell wall of the *Candida* organism until it dissolves. The FDA approved the switch of Femstat 3 from prescription to over-the-counter status in December 1996 and that for Vagistat in February 1997. The other products have been available over the counter for a few years.

Despite the effectiveness of these medications, the recurrence rate of the infection can be very high *following* treatment. Almost half of all patients will experience a repeat episode after just four weeks. In addition, these drugs have a range of side-effects. Common but minor side-effects include headache as well as vaginal burning, infection, itching, and inflammation. More rare side-effects include rash; sore throat; abdominal pain; nasal inflammation; painful urination or frequent urination at night; swelling of the vulva; vaginal dryness, irritation, pain, or discharge; and pain during sexual intercourse.

In light of this wide range of side-effects, you might wonder whether taking an antifungal drug is worth it. Certainly, when the side-effects of a medication are just as bad or worse than the condition itself, a quick cost/benefit analysis will tell you that no, it's not worth it. Even the fact that the recurrence rate of infection typically goes up after treatment should make anyone think twice about using these drugs. Even so, before you decide anything, be sure to talk to your health care provider.

Another point to consider is that the FDA requires all over-the-counter products for treating yeast infections to carry the following warning:

If you experience vaginal yeast infections frequently (they recur within a two-month period) or if you have vaginal yeast infections that do not clear up easily with proper treatment, you should see your doctor promptly to determine the cause and receive proper medical care.

The reason this warning was issued is that having recurrent yeast infections or difficult-to-cure yeast infections may indicate an underlying immunological problem. This would make the individual much more susceptible to so-called *opportunistic diseases*, which are always ready to take advantage of a weakened immune system. In some cases, the problem may be life threatening—in the case of developing AIDS, for instance. Needless to say, this product warning should be taken quite seriously.

Again, when you have a yeast infection for the first time, you should visit your doctor to be diagnosed. Also ask him or her which product may be best for you, and discuss the advantages of the different forms the products come in (for instance, vaginal suppositories versus creams with special applicators) along with their known side-effects.

Whatever product you use, carefully read any warnings on the product's labeling and follow all directions regarding its use. Your symptoms will usually improve within a few days of treatment. Even so, you should continue using the medication for the number of days directed, even if you no longer have symptoms. Finally, if you are sexually active, your partner should also be treated, as yeast infections can be spread through intercourse.

WHAT IS THE PROBIOTIC SOLUTION?

Until recently, the imbalance of organisms in a yeast infection was seen as a *result* of the infection. But now, it's understood that the imbalance of organisms can *cause* the infection, not the other way around. The only way to solve this imbalance is to address the level of probiotics in the urogenital system (UGS), which can be done in a number of ways.

First of all, let's consider what the good organisms in the UGS usually do to keep the bad organisms in check. They do pretty much the same things they do in other parts of the body: They produce a number of compounds, some of which are natural antibiotics that directly attack the bad guys and leave the good guys alone.

The good organisms also lower the pH of the UGS. This is important because the pathogenic (bad) organisms do not like to have as low a pH as the probiotic (good) organisms do. The probiotics naturally produce acids, such as lactic acid, and hence are called *lactic acid bacteria*. Their very presence inhibits the growth of the pathogenics. The bad bacteria, in effect, find themselves surrounded by acid, from which they have little or no protection, and they die.

The probiotics also produce hydrogen peroxide. In the UGS, hydrogen peroxide does what it normally does when used to clean a wound: It kills bacteria. The pathogenic bacteria are especially vulnerable, whereas the probiotics tend to be more resistant. As described elsewhere, this is a game of numbers. The type of bacteria present in the greatest number win. This is one of the reasons it makes sense to pulse with probiotics initially and overwhelm the enemy, the bad bacteria. (The *Brudnak method* for pulsing and rotating probiotics will be discussed more in Chapter 10 on delivery systems.)

Given these benefits, probiotics can be used successfully in the treatment of yeast infections. One way to do so is to eat yogurt that contains active, live organisms. This has been a traditional remedy of sorts for some time, and we will discuss it in more detail later in this section. Yogurt can also be used as a suppository. In fact, in Europe, suppositories are available that contain lyophilized *acidophilus*. They are produced by freeze-drying and then encapsulating high numbers of lactic acid bacteria. The suppository is inserted into the target location (say, the vagina), where the capsule dissolves and releases the probiotics. The probiotics then implant and grow.

This is exactly what happens naturally in the body when a person is healthy. Probiotics grow and flourish inside the vagina and other parts of the UGS, keeping the pathogenic organisms at bay. We all have probiotic organisms in and on our *mucous membranes*, which line the passages and cavities of the body that directly contact either air (such as the vagina) or the food we eat (such as the colon). And when an imbalance occurs, for whatever reason, the number of probiotics drops off, causing a rise in the pH and an opening up of the attachment sites where pathogenic organisms can hook on and start to grow.

Let's look specifically at the infection that results from *Candida albicans*, which is the most common type of yeast infection. It's known that lactic acid can inhibit *Candida albicans*, but exactly how this happens is unclear. It seems as though some sort of balancing act is going on among three different players: the lactic acid bacteria, the *Candida albicans*, and the level of carbohydrates present. We have talked about the first two, but what is the role of carbohydrates?

Carbohydrates come in different forms, but they all share the same basic chemical makeup. What they look like is not really important, but for the sake of simplicity, let's just say they are all sugar. That sugar is actually a combination of two sugars called *glucose* and *fructose*. Glucose is what is commonly referred to as *blood sugar*. Most sugars must be broken down to or converted into glucose to be utilized effectively. This is true of body cells, bacterial cells, and yeast cells. Almost all types of life love sugar! And the simpler it is, the less energy it takes to break it down, and the faster it can be eaten and used as food.

How much sugar is present in any part of the body, at any given time, is usually tightly controlled because microorganisms have the potential to misuse large amounts to further their own growth. This is what causes a yeast infection. In fact, when yeast or bacteria are grown in the lab, some sugar is always thrown in to speed up how fast the cells will multiply. When bacteria are fed a pure glucose solution, they are in "hog heaven," so to speak. When this is done with probiotics, the sugars are called *prebiotics* as long as they are selective and do not stimulate the growth of pathogenic organisms. Glucose is not a prebiotic because even the bad guys can use it.

Sugar can be overly abundant in the body, making it prone to yeast infections, for several different reasons. For instance, a diet that is high in sugar and carbohydrates can support the growth of yeast and similar organisms. Conditions in which the body does not utilize sugar properly, such as diabetes, can also lead to extraordinarily high levels of sugars being present. Diebetics will actually excrete large amounts of sugar in their urine. Again, this creates an environment that is very favorable to the growth of bacteria and yeast: namely, one that is warm, moist, and sugary.

As mentioned already, yogurt has been used for many years to treat yeast infections. The clinical results have been mixed: sometimes good and sometimes nothing special. One of the problems with using yogurt, as verified by research, is that not all dairy products contain *Lactobacillus*, which is thought to be the most important organism for treating yeast infections. Also, those products that do contain it may contain only low levels of probiotics that are actually alive and viable. To use yogurt successfully as a treatment, it's important to find a manufacturer that is reputable and knows how to distribute and handle these products. More specifically, the manufacturer needs to know how *not* to handle them!

The handling of probiotics can be even more important than the actual growing of them, which is called *fermentation*. Probiotics are extremely susceptible to a set of conditions that are collectively called *variables*: temperature, water, and food, for instance. If these variables are not all strictly controlled during fermentation and handling, the viability of the probiotics will be drastically altered—and always in a bad way. For this reason, it's vital to optimize the growth conditions of probiotics during their manufacture. (Very few companies really know how to do this well, which I will address more in Chapter 10 on delivery systems.)

Again, what's most important is that *Lactobacillus* and *Bifidobacteria* be present because the two primary organisms found in yogurt—*Streptococcus thermophilus* and *Lactobacillus bulgaricus*—are transient organisms. That is, they don't implant in the GI tract. In order for them to be effective in treating yeast infections, they must be continually supplied in large numbers to the GI tract and backed up by a *Lactobacillus* organism, such as LA-5.

To recap, when pathogenic bacteria are present in large numbers, you want to get them out fast. That's the purpose of pulsing with probiotics. Suppositories are especially effective, as extremely high numbers of probiotics can be delivered directly to the afflicted area. It's also effective to combine the probiotics with other foods that can assist in the fight against the bad bacteria. In particular, the use of cranberry products is a popular treatment for urinary tract infections (UTIs), which can be either bacterial or yeast infections.

The GI tract is a dynamic system, in which things change all the time. As part of this change, the resident bacteria, both good and bad, are constantly attaching and detaching. If the bad bacteria outnumber the good, the result is disease or infection. This happens because the good bacteria—the probiotics—cannot make a "beachhead" on which to take hold and shift the balance in their favor.

Cranberry powder, which has an antiadhesion factor, can prevent the binding of bacteria. So when it's added to a probiotic bacteria formulation, it allows that initial beachhead to be established. The proliferation of bad bacteria is counteracted by the cranberry, which causes more of the bad bacteria to detach than would normally be the case. This frees up space on the intestinal surface for the good bacteria to attach to and get to work.

Granted, cranberry powder may have a similar effect on some of the good bacteria, causing them to detach. This, however, has never been demonstrated. Keep in mind how many good bacteria are being added back into the GI tract through probiotic supplementation—billions, in most cases. Adding this large number of probiotic organisms allows the equilibrium of the system to shift back in favor of the good guys. Moreover, cranberry powder is *not* 100 percent efficient. It does not cause all the bacteria to detach but simply opens up spaces in the colonies of the intestines to which the good bacteria can attach. Given these benefits, combination products, such as probiotic/cranberry blends, likely represent the future of probiotic products.

As researchers continue to study the use of probiotics to treat conditions such as yeast infections, the growth of knowledge in this area will be enormous. Moreover, the likely result will be the increased use of probiotics in this and other applications. Not only are probiotics safe and effective, but they don't have the wide-ranging side-effects that many over-the-counter drugs have. It's already commonplace in Europe and Japan to treat yeast infections with probiotics, which means it's just a matter of time until this is done in the United States.

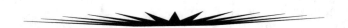

CHAPTER 8

Why Probiotics Promise Relief from Irritable Bowel Syndrome

WHAT IS IRRITABLE BOWEL SYNDROME?

Irritable bowel syndrome (IBS) is the most common gastrointestinal (GI) disorder. The symptoms include crampy pain, gassiness, bloating, and changes in bowel habits. Some people with IBS have constipation (that is, difficult or infrequent bowel movements); others have diarrhea (that is, frequent and loose stools, often with an urgent need to move the bowels); and some people have both alternately. Others with IBS have a cramping urge to move the bowels but cannot do so; others pass mucus with their bowel movements.

In diagnosing IBS, it's important to realize that what is considered *normal* bowel function varies from person to person. It may range from as many as three stools a day to as few as three a week. In addition, a normal bowel movement is one that is formed but not hard, contains no blood, and is passed without cramps or pain. Bleeding, fever, weight loss, and persistent severe pain are *not* symptoms of IBS but may indicate other problems.

Over the years, IBS has been called by many names—*colitis, mucous colitis, spastic colon, spastic bowel,* and *functional bowel disease*—but most of these terms are inaccurate. *Colitis,* for instance, involves inflammation of the large intestine (or colon). While inflammation is a symptom of IBS, IBS does not cause inflammation, and so it shouldn't be confused with another disorder, *ulcerative colitis.*

IBS causes a great deal of discomfort and distress, but it does not usually cause permanent harm to the intestines. Similarly, IBS does not lead to intestinal bleeding of the bowel or to serious diseases such as cancer. In fact, doctors call IBS a *functional disorder* because there is no sign of disease when the colon is examined. Nutritional deficiencies and anorexia may be observed in some cases, however.

When left untreated, IBS is very serious, usually resulting in surgery. Surgery is performed to remove the part of the colon that has become infected through constant irritation and weakened immune functioning. After surgery, the colon must be allowed time to heal, so the patient temporarily wears an external bag to collect the body's waste. This is rare with IBS, however.

For many people, IBS is just a mild annoyance, but for others, it can be disabling. In severe cases, people may be unable to go to social events, to travel even short distances, or even to go to work. Most people, however, are able to control their symptoms through managing diet and stress and through taking prescription medication.

WHAT CAUSES IRRITABLE BOWEL SYNDROME?

Doctors have not been able to find an organic cause for IBS, so it's often thought to result from emotional conflict and stress. While conflict and stress do likely worsen the symptoms of IBS, research suggests that other factors also are important. In particular, it's been discovered that the colon muscle of a person with IBS begins to spasm after only mild stimulation.

How is the colon supposed to work? The colon, which is about 3-5 feet long, is actually part of the large intestine; it connects the small intestine with the rectum and the anus. The major function of the colon is to absorb water and salts from the digestive products that enter from the small intestine. An estimated 2 quarts of liquid matter enter the colon from the small intestine each day. This material may remain there for several days until most of the fluid and salts are absorbed into the body. The stool then passes through the colon by a pattern of movements to the left side of the colon, where it's stored until a bowel movement occurs.

Ordinary events such as eating and distention (that is, bloating) from gas and other materials can cause the colon to overreact in the person with IBS. Certain medicines and foods may also trigger spasms in certain people. Sometimes, the spasm delays the passage of the stool, leading to constipation. Chocolate, dairy products, and large amounts of alcohol are frequent offenders. And while caffeine causes loose stools in many people, it's more likely to affect those with IBS. Researchers also have found that women with IBS may have more symptoms during the menstrual period, suggesting that reproductive hormones may somehow stimulate the colon.

HOW IS IRRITABLE BOWEL SYNDROME TREATED?

Irritable bowel syndrome is managed primarily through dietary means. For some people, that might mean watching their caloric intake or following a stricter food plan, perhaps avoiding foods that seem troublesome (dairy products, for instance). Avoiding certain drugs, such as antidiarrheals and osteoporosis medications (unless they are prescribed), may also help relieve the symptoms of IBS. In more severe cases, IBS might be managed through consuming a liquid diet or taking fiber supplements.

Managing stress is also an important element in treating IBS. While the exact relationship between stress and IBS isn't well understood, it is known that stress plays an important role. Part of the problem may be that you've diverged from your regular lifestyle—what you eat, what you drink, how much and how well you sleep, how much exercise you get, and so on. Think about how traveling can affect bowel function, especially long-distance traveling, like going overseas. Most people are constipated upon arrival and can remain so for several days, even weeks, unless they take something. Also think about how many stressful situations involving sitting—for instance, working long hours at your desk or sitting in a hospital waiting room. Regardless of whether we understand *why* stress has this effect on us, we must recognize that it *does!*

A few prescription drugs can also be used to treat IBS, including sulphasalazine, olsalazine, balsalazide, and tegaserod. Interestingly, these drugs have very specific effects in terms of the symptoms they are able to control and even how they work in men versus women. Tegaserod, for example, is a selective serotonin receptor agonist that's been found effective in treating IBS in women who have *constipation* as the main symptom. (This drug is similar to the SSRI-class drugs like Prozac, which are used to treat depression. Both drugs have the effect of leaving more serotonin in the system.) Interesting, Tegaserod has not been found effective in treating IBS in women who have *diarrhea* as the major symptom, nor has it been shown to work at all in *men* with IBS, which suggests that what causes this condition varies greatly. Given these differences in effectiveness, it's very important that someone with IBS sees a doctor and gets an *individual* diagnosis and treatment recommendation. More specifically, taking someone else's IBS medication is a bad idea. Prescription drug treatment is never a "one size fits all" proposition!

Some over-the-counter products are also available at drugstores for treating irritable bowel syndrome. For instance, products like Gas-X and Phazyme will help relieve the pressure that comes from having gas, and antacids will help, as well, if acid buildup is what's causing the gas. A whole range of laxatives are also available, from the very powerful Ex-Lax to the less powerful fiber products and herbal preparations, such as Senna.

Just keep in mind that even the most mild of these products can have an undesirable cumulative effect, especially with ongoing use. For instance, if you use a laxative on a regular basis, even at just a low level, your body may become physically dependent on it for proper functioning. In effect, your body will figure out that it doesn't have to work so hard to get the job done, so it will scale back its efforts. Similarly, if you are a chronic user of antidiarrheal products, your body may get used to having help and lose its natural ability to handle excess water. Most over-the-counter products for treating IBS are sold as *nutritional supplements,* rather than *medications,* because supplement manufacturers are not legally allowed to treat diseases or disorders; rather, they can only support natural body functioning. The result is that these products typically have odd names, which makes it difficult for the average consumer to find them. In fact, a search for "Irritable Bowel Syndrome" on the website drugstore.com turned up only one product, which was intended to control the water level in the colon. Other useful products are likely indexed under other topics, since their manufacturers can't say outright that they treat IBS. But without knowing that (let alone what other topics to look for), you wouldn't have any luck finding an over-the-counter treatment.

So, let me mention several nutritional supplements that might help with IBS (and of course, we'll talk about using probiotics in the next section). The brand Basic Nutrition, sold by the massive health food store GNC, has a product called Magnesium (as Magnesium Oxide and Magnesium Gluconate) that is marketed for use in treating IBS. Senna, the herbal product mentioned earlier, is also effective. Finally, the enzyme *Alpha galactosidase* may be useful in that it can digest some of the common carbohydrates from which gas is produced.

In sum, let me say that over-the-counter products have their place when used according to directions and in *moderation.* Regardless, you should consult your health care provider and get his or her recommendations for medications and other treatment approaches.

Surgery is the final option in treating IBS and should only be considered after all other options have been exhausted. In fact, very few people end up having surgery to treat IBS. The "good news" is that the surgery does seem to work; the "bad news" is that it is incredibly invasive and dramatic. Nonetheless, there are times when surgery is necessary, and it's conceivable that waiting too long to take this step could cause more serious and even permanent damage to other systems of the body. Again, anyone with IBS should see his or her doctor and learn about the full range of treatments available.

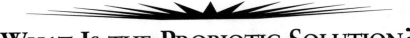

WHAT IS THE PROBIOTIC SOLUTION?

Again, exactly what causes IBS is unknown, which is perhaps why the traditional treatments take only a patchwork approach. That is, they address just the symptoms, not what's happening in terms of the biology of the gut. Probiotics, on the other hand, can beneficially and permanently change the functionality of the gut—and that's exciting!

So, what *is* happening in the gut? For some reason, the gastrointestinal (GI) tract gets overtaken by pathogenic (or bad) bacteria. A variety of these bacteria can be involved; regardless, it's the large number of them in the gut that causes the problem. By themselves, they can cause all the symptoms associated with IBS.

Taking high doses of probiotics when you have a condition such as IBS has several effects—all of them positive! First, the good bacteria will physically push out some of the bad bacteria. Second, some of the bad bacteria will be killed by the natural antibiotics that the probiotics will produce. Third, the probiotics will stimulate the body to produce antibodies of its own, which will not only attack the bacteria but also help regulate the body's overactive immune response to the bad bacteria. Finally, the probiotics will create or condition their environment such that they will stabilize the pH of the GI tract to a normal level. When that happens, the pathogenic bacteria will naturally be inhibited because they don't like that sort of pH. (Remember, the pH is simply a relative indication of the amount of acid in any particular place—in this case, the GI tract.)

Using probiotics to reduce the number of bad bacteria in the GI tract also has another interesting effect: There will be fewer bad bacteria dying. Believe it or not, this is a good thing! When bad bacteria die, their cellular bodies break up and release the highly toxic elements that made them bad in the first place. So, even when they are dead, these bacteria can damage the body. In fact, this often causes what's known as a *healing crisis* in someone who starts a successful program of probiotics therapy. While the bad bacteria are being killed, the person can initially feel a bit worse. That feeling usually goes away after a few days, but it can last a couple of weeks if the process is not immediate.

Enzymatic insufficiencies also play a role in IBS. When the body has a shortage of certain enzymes, it has difficulty digesting food. By supplementing with high doses of probiotics, the body gets not only those beneficial organisms but also all the really good enzymes that are active in those cells. Having all these enzymes will help digest the extra food materials that the body's own enzymes are having trouble with. It's vital that high doses of probiotics be used because the bacteria in the gut have most of the same enzymes that the body has.

For instance, the use of an enzyme product called *Beano* is extremely popular for relieving the intestinal gas that's typically produced from eating beans. The reason this product works is that it contains an enzyme that digests the special sugars found in beans. Those sugars are very difficult for the body to digest because it doesn't produce the particular enzyme necessary for that digestion. (Interestingly, that particular enzyme is naturally found at high levels in some probiotics.) When the sugars in beans aren't broken down, they come in contact with the bad bacteria in the GI tract, which are present in high numbers in someone with IBS. As it happens, bad bacteria really like those sugars! In fact, they like them so much that they eat as many of the sugars as they can. And when they do, one of the results is gas.

Now, anyone who has ever had that sort of gas knows that it can be really troubling, in several respects. Physically, the condition is at least uncomfortable and sometimes downright painful. In extreme cases, the pain can last for days. The reason for this intense pain is that the intestines are lined with millions of nerve cells. Actually, the intestines are sometimes referred to as "the second brain" because the vast array of nerve cells found there is similar to that in the brain. The nerve cells in the intestines can transmit pain impulses, and that's how we know when something is wrong down there.

The probiotic *Lactobacillus plantarum* has been used successfully to decrease the pain and flatulence associated with IBS. Typically, a reasonable dosage of around 40 billion is used (that is, 400 milliliters of a 100,000,000 organisms/milliliter). That sounds like an awful lot, but it really isn't. Consider that a single serving of fresh, homemade yogurt can have 100s of billions of organisms.

Again, while IBS does not cause inflammation, inflammation is one of the *symptoms* of IBS (or at the very least, it may be present when someone has IBS). Probiotics can be effective in this area, too, as a number of them seem to decrease inflammation, if that's a concern. It's commonly accepted that probiotics do this through their ability to induce the human body to produce *antibodies*. Put simply, the body makes many different products that are important for an immune response, including antibodies. Antibodies come in several varieties, each with unique properties. One called *IgA* is very interesting because it not only acts like a typical antibody—that is, binding to bad materials that enter the body—but it also has a feedback function that helps reduce the immune response. It sort of says to the body, "Hey, I've got things under control." IgA also calls off another antibody that has been implicated in such conditions as diabetes and allergic reactions.

Again, probiotics don't just break down a lot of the food we eat; in addition, they contribute to the health and well-being of the body's own cells. Another example of how probiotics do this is that they provide a physical barrier for the *colonocytes*, or the cells lining the GI, in general. When there is an overgrowth of pathogenic bacteria in the GI, a lot of these bacteria produce compounds that are highly toxic to the body. Some of them produce proteins called *peptides*, some of which can have a devastating effect. These toxins can cross the natural barrier of the body (that is, the cells lining the GI) and enter the body. When probiotics are ingested to populate or repopulate the GI tract to a normal level, they can prevent the growth of these pathogenic organisms.

To assist in treating IBS, a number of probiotic products are worth looking at. Some companies produce high-potency, documented strains that will be effective. Since many different types of probiotics are found in the human gut, it's advisable to look for a product that contains several different organisms and 20 to 40 billion organisms per dose. Taking one capsule, several times a day, is sufficient.

HLN has such a product, EnteroHealth, which contains over 40 billion organisms per capsule at the time it's manufactured. (And to HLN's credit, they only claim that the product contains 30 billion organisms, so as not to overstate the number that are likely alive at the time of purchase or eventual use.) EnteroHealth offers a comprehensive replacement of six well-recognized, well-researched, and clinically effective probiotic strains to support and enhance GI health. In addition, these six strains are unequaled in strain purity and identity and have outstanding long-term viability and stability. This extraordinary supplement is also guaranteed to be free of casein/milk, wheat, corn, yeast, sucrose, starch, and artificial colors—all of which can have negative effects on both probiotic and human health. Finally, what I find to be the strongest selling point of EnteroHealth is that all the strains and the product itself have undergone the MAKTech process of qualification. (We'll talk more about this process in Chapter 10.) Again, it's absolutely vital to purchase reputable, qualified products.

Picking a good *prebiotic* (such as glucosamine HCl, Lactulose, FOS, or Inulin) is important, too, so that the probiotics have something to live on. The probiotics can eat a lot of the food we eat, but they do prefer some things over others. It's great when the prebiotic is supplied in the same capsule as the probiotics, because the food will be right there when they are moistened in the body and able to grow.

One company, Klaire Laboratories, is doing clinical, blinded studies on the use of probiotics to treat IBS. When I contacted Dr. Jeff Mersky, vice president of Klaire Laboratories, he had this to say about Klaire's research:

Of course, Klaire is known as the first in the nutritional industry to introduce dairy-free and maltodextrin-free friendly bacteria, and we've been a leader in this field since 1983. Because of our track record and integrity as a company, we are asked to participate in university-based studies. Presently, we have been involved with the University of Kansas and Stanford University to study the effects of probiotics on irritable bowel syndrome. Dr. Jeannie Drisko of Kansas reports that 20 patients were used in this NIH-granted, year-long study. They are patients who have never known anything but diarrhea their entire adult lives, and they were given up as incurable by their GI doctors. The study, completed in January [2003], had preliminary findings of a cure for 16 out of 20 patients. This is quite remarkable and has stirred quite a bit of excitement at the Kansas Gastroenterology Department. Dr. Drisko plans on using this data to secure grant money for a full-blown double-blind study in the near future.

Klaire has also been asked to participate in a double-blind study involving patients who have organ transplants and are given immuno-suppressive drugs, which always cause diarrhea. The Swedish Hospital in Seattle, Washington, has received grant money for a two-year study involving our probiotics for the possibilities of controlling the side effects of bowel problems with organ transplants. Having the confidence of the scientific community and offering the best probiotic products available to the clinician and public is what Klaire is all about.

Talking with Dr. Mersky convinced me that the people at Klaire Laboratories know their products and their science, which is the best sales endorsement I can think of. With Klaire Labs, you can trust in the quality of their products. If you or a loved one has IBS or a similar condition and is interested in support, I suggest contacting Dr. Mersky and his team and asking for more information. (See the Resources section at the end of the book for contact information.) I'm sure they will happily assist you.

The use of probiotics seems to be the most promising approach to treating IBS because it does more than just treat the symptoms. Getting inside the gut is what's needed to provide relief to the countless people who have this condition—the most common of all GI disorders.

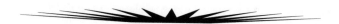

CHAPTER 9

How Probiotics Can Help Alleviate the Symptoms of Down Syndrome

WHAT IS DOWN SYNDROME?

Down syndrome (DS) is a congenital type of mental retardation that involves moderate to severe mental impairment along with a range of distinctive physical traits. These traits vary considerably from one individual to another and may include a flat facial profile; a sloping forehead; an upward slant to the eyes; a short neck; low-set ears; small ear canals; white or light-gray spots at the outer edge of the iris (called *Brushfield spots*); short, broad hands; a single, deep transverse crease on the palm of the hand; and a generally dwarflike physique.

Many of these features are readily apparent in a newborn baby with DS, such that the attending physician will recognize the condition. However, a child with DS may not possess all of these features, and some of these features can be found among the general population.

How can a diagnosis of Down syndrome be confirmed? The doctor will request a blood test called a *chromosomal karyotype*. It involves growing the cells from the baby's blood for about two weeks and then examining the chromosomes under a microscopic to determine if extra material from chromosome number 21 is present. An individual with DS has an extra chromosome—usually, number 21 or 22.

Down syndrome was named in 1866 by John Langdon Hydon Down, who had observed two classical clinical manifestations: abnormal coordination and abnormal circulation. Since Down's time, a large collection of maladies have been associated with DS, many of them congenital. People with DS are at greater risk for having congenital heart defects and kidney defects and for developing visual impairments, upper-respiratory infections, and leukemia. Researchers have also discovered a link between DS and Alzheimer's disease, although the exact nature of that link is still unclear.

Of particular interest in this book is the wide range of abnormalities commonly found in people with DS that involve the gastrointestinal (GI) tract, including the following: duodenal atresia (that is, there is a closure or lack of duodenum), pancreatic insufficiency (not enough digestive enzymes are produced), imperforated anus (the anus is closed or sealed), and enlarged colon (this causes a buildup of waste materials). And certain other conditions may *appear* to be GI in nature and mistakenly treated as such—for instance, pulmonic stenosis, which involves narrowing of the lung passages.

These various GI conditions are often diagnosed due to the individual's failure to put on weight or sometimes the reverse, which is the tendency toward obesity. The individual can appear hypometabolic and experience extremes across his or her lifetime. In infancy, he or she may have poor nutrition and difficulty putting on weight. But then in adolescence and beyond, weight may become an issue because the individual tends to put on too much.

As mentioned already, a huge proportion of people with DS also seem to get Alzheimer's disease. Understanding why will involve examining the relationship between what's happening in the gut and in the brain in both of these diseases. Interestingly, neurological development seems inseparable from GI maturation. If there's a problem with the gut, it's almost always reflected in the development of the brain.

A very high proportion of people with DS also have what is known as *celiac disease*, which is an intestinal malabsorption syndrome. Celiac disease involves diarrhea and malnutrition and can be characterized by poor growth and weight loss. Again, this is a GI dysfunction. Of the DS population, 1 in 6 to 1 in 14 has celiac disease (compared to 1 in 300 of the general population).

In the final stage of DS, the individual can no longer walk or feed himself or herself and is thus bedridden. A neurologic examination may show abnormal nose, grasp, and suck reflexes along with bilateral extensor plantar reflexes, which results in an irregular gait or walk. Death usually results from malnutrition, sepsis (a toxic condition resulting from the spread of bacteria or their products from a focus of infection), or aspiration pneumonia (in which foreign matter is inhaled into the lungs).

Given all of these health problems, the life expectancy of someone with DS is well below normal—around the age of 50. However, most individuals with DS are capable of leading productive lives, given the appropriate programming and social support.

WHAT CAUSES DOWN SYNDROME?

To understand why Down syndrome occurs, you must understand the structure and function of the human chromosome. The human body is made of cells, and all cells contain *chromosomes*, structures that transmit genetic information. Most cells of the human body contain 23 pairs of chromosomes, half of which are inherited from each parent. Only the human reproductive cells—that is, the sperm cells in males and the ova in females—have 23 *individual* chromosomes, not pairs. Scientists identify these chromosome pairs as the *XX pair*, present in females, and the *XY pair*, present in males, and number them 1 through 22, plus the sex pair.

When the reproductive cells, the sperm and ovum, combine at fertilization, the fertilized egg that results contains 23 chromosome pairs. A fertilized egg that will develop into a female contains chromosome pairs 1 through 22 plus the XX pair. A fertilized egg that will develop into a male contains chromosome pairs 1 through 22 plus the XY pair. When the fertilized egg contains extra material from chromosome number 21, the result is Down syndrome.

Most of the time, the occurrence of DS is due to a random event that occurred during formation of the reproductive cells—the ovum or the sperm. As far as scientists know, DS cannot be attributed to any behavioral activity of the parents or to environmental factors.

Researchers have found, however, that the incidence of Down syndrome increases with maternal age. The likelihood that a woman under 30 who becomes pregnant will have a baby with DS is less than 1 in 1,000, but for a woman who become pregnant at age 35, that incidence increases to 1 in 400. By age 42, the chance is 1 in 60 that a pregnant woman will have a baby with DS, and by age 49, the chance is 1 in 12.

Why is maternal age so important? As a woman ages, there is a dramatic increase in the likelihood that one of her reproductive cells will contain an extra copy of chromosome 21. Therefore, an older mother is more likely than a younger mother to have a baby with DS. But using maternal age alone will not detect three out of four of the pregnancies that result in Down syndrome. Of the total population, older mothers have fewer babies. This means that about 75 percent of the babies with DS are born to younger women simply because younger women have more babies than older women. Yet the age issue is still significant. While only about 9 percent of the total number of pregnancies each year occur in women 35 years or older, about 25 percent of the babies with DS are born to women in this age group. Regardless of maternal age, however, the probability that a woman will have another child with Down syndrome in a subsequent pregnancy is only about 1 percent.

Given the relationship between maternal age and DS, many specialists recommend that women who become pregnant at age 35 or older undergo prenatal testing for this condition. This screening involves a relatively simple, noninvasive test that examines a drop of the mother's blood and measures the levels of three markers for Down syndrome:

serum alpha feto-protein (MSAFP), chorionic gonadotropin (hCG), and unconjugated estriol (uE3). While these measurements do not provide a definitive test for Down syndrome, a lower MSAFP value, a lower uE3 level, and an elevated hCG level usually suggest an increased likelihood of the fetus having Down syndrome, and additional diagnostic testing may be desired.

HOW IS DOWN SYNDROME TREATED?

There is no medical cure for Down syndrome. However, with early detection, many of the other conditions that appear in people with DS, such as heart defects and gastrointestinal problems, can be corrected. Doing so will not only improve the individual's quality of life but will increase his or her life expectancy, as well.

Early intervention is also important in the area of education. Beginning as early as infancy, it's important to provide activities that stimulate the child's sensory, motor, and cognitive skills. Research has found that children with DS who participate in an intensive preschool education program score higher on intelligence tests (that is, usually in the "mildly retarded" range) than children with DS who do not participate in this type of program.

The parents and family of a child with Down syndrome may also help enhance his or her development. By being closely involved in the child's school activities, a parent or other family member might recognize individual abilities—for instance, that the child tends to learn better through visual than auditory means. A child with DS may have a better understanding than his or her language skills indicate. Finally, enjoying loving, caring relationships with parents and family members can have a positive effect on the child's emotional development.

The parents of children with Down syndrome may find it worthwhile to belong to parent-support groups, which are available in most cities and on the Internet, as well. Sharing knowledge and resources, along with emotions and experiences, can be enormously beneficial to these parents.

WHAT IS THE PROBIOTIC SOLUTION?

As noted earlier, people with Down syndrome often have a variety of gastrointestinal (GI) disorders, including pancreatic insufficiency, enlarged colon, and celiac disease. None of these disorders is exclusive to people with DS, and in an otherwise healthy individual, the symptoms of these disorders would be more annoying than anything else. But for someone with Down syndrome, these conditions are often more severe, in part, because they often occur together. What's more, the person with DS will likely find it difficult to understand why he or she has GI problems, and it may be overwhelming for him or her to have several or all of these conditions at the same time.

The cumulative effect of having one or more of these GI problems can best be understood by briefly reviewing how the GI tract works. To begin, think of the body as a "hollow tube." The tube starts at the mouth, where food is put in, and runs down through the body to the anus, where waste is expelled. The *gastrointestinal tract* is that part of the tube running from the stomach to the anus, which is where most of digestion occurs. The GI tract is essentially the *intestines*—small and large—and runs about 25 feet in most humans.

The first part of the *small intestine* (about 20 feet long) is called the *duodenum*, and it connects the intestines to the stomach. The other parts of the small intestine are the *jejunum* and *ileum*. Next is the *large intestine* (3—5 feet long), which includes the *cecum*, *colon*, and *rectum*. The *anus* is the actual opening at the end of the rectum, where waste exits the body. Each of the sections of the GI tract is made up of different cells and tissues and thus has a different environment (or pH) and a different purpose.

Different probiotics are found at different locations throughout the GI tract. In fact, there are more probiotic organisms in the human GI tract than there are human cells in the human body—and that's a lot of cells! All of these probiotics are constantly supplying enzymes to assist in the digestion of food that has been passed on from the stomach. Yet probiotics perform many, many important functions for the human host beyond digestion. In short, when probiotics are malfunctioning or absent, then disease sets in.

We are used to thinking that when we eat a cookie, it passes through the body as a cookie (or maybe as a ground-up cookie), but it's much more complicated than that. As that cookie makes its way, each portion of the GI tract acts on it and then passes it on to the next portion in the state most favorable for that next portion to do its job. It's like an assembly line, with each section having a certain job to do.

The trouble occurs when one or more sections don't do their jobs. For instance, the duodenum is where a great deal of metabolic activity happens. It's where the stomach empties into the small intestine and the food gets neutralized by digestive enzymes. The pancreas is responsible for producing a large amount of these enzymes, and it supplies them into this area of the GI tract. In doing so, it raises the pH of the duodenum, which means it increases the alkalinity there.

Given all this activity, the duodenum has cells that are designed to handle large swings in pH. But if those pH swings take too long at any given level, then the cells' ability to resist damage can be overcome and the cells might die. If the pH stays too low, for instance, the probiotics will be less likely to survive and thus not contribute their enzymes; moreover, the enzymes that are there won't function as well. (This is because all enzymes function best at certain temperatures and pHs—namely, the normal pH of the body at that given location.) If the pH is not corrected, the body cells will die off, too. And to further worsen the situation, the lower-acid pH materials will be passed on to subsequent areas of the intestines and kill off the cells there (that is, both the probiotics and the human body cells).

When the cells along the GI are damaged by the improper processing of food and nutrients, as occurs in people with DS, they become inflamed and subject to immunological activities. Basically, there is an influx of immune cells. Also, as the food processing is altered, a lot of gas may be produced and cause swelling of the intestines. This is very typical for people with DS.

As mentioned, when there is a dysfunction in any section of the GI, it eventually spreads from the small intestine to the large intestine and ultimately to the colon. Usually, all the absorption of nutrients happens in the small intestine, but that won't be the case if there is a massive influx of immune cells there, trying to fight the inflammation. The immune cells not only make compounds that can retard absorption, but they also physically get in the way of the cells and don't let the nutrients pass. And even though it might seem that the presence of gas should help the nutrients get absorbed, it doesn't. Ultimately, certain molecules (namely, bad bacteria) will get absorbed that you just don't want in the body.

Let's talk a little more about the immune cells getting in the way. For normal functionality, the absorbing cells of the body need to be in close proximity to each other. If they are swollen and pushed away from one another, then they can't "chat" back and forth. Cells are actually very social and like to talk with their neighbors to make sure everyone is happy; if they don't get positive feedback from one another, they get very insecure and clam up. When this happens, they not only stop talking but stop absorbing, as well. Large substances, like bacteria, may get by them, but that's basically because of the increased spaces around the cells, not because the cells are absorbing them.

With this loss of sites of absorption in the GI tract, the probiotics get wiped out. That will affect the digestion of food and also the movement of the intestines. Probiotics assist with having a bowel movement, so when they are dead, things grind to a halt. And when there is a blockage in the colon, all kinds of bad things happen. Specifically, material builds up, pushing the cells outward and expanding the size of the colon. The intestine is literally stretched out, and this has been observed clinically in people with DS.

What can be done? The first thing that's needed is to correct the pancreatic insufficiency in the small intestine, which is one of the hallmarks of DS. The pancreas itself cannot be fixed, but most of the enzymes that have been lost can be replaced by taking large numbers of probiotics. In fact, products have been designed specifically based on knowledge of the organisms normally found functioning in certain areas of the GI tract. One such product, AdvoCare's Biotic Buddies, contains both *Lactobacillus acidophilus* and *Bifidobacterium bifidum*, which are naturally found in the small intestine and the colon, respectively. Plus, this product tastes so good that even the most finicky kids will gobble it up!

Mostly *Lactobacilli* are found in the upper GI, such as the duodenum, the part of the small intestine closest to the stomach. Large doses (that is, containing 40 to 100 billion organisms each) can be used safely and effectively. HLN's Gently Rotate has over 40 billion organisms per capsule and can be used as one element in the *Brudnak method* of pulsing and rotating. A dose of Gently Rotate can serve as the "rotation" element, which means it would follow a "pulse" element of high doses of one or two organisms, typically targeting either the colon or the small intestine. Once favorable results have been achieved, a "maintenance" product can be introduced that supplies a lower number of organisms (1 to 4 billion) but of a mixed variety. This final supplementation is more representative of a normal GI tract and thus serves to stabilize it.

In fact, doses even higher than 40 billion organisms have been used without any side-effects. Consider that if yogurt is freshly fermented, the number of live bacteria it contains can be well over 100 billion per milliliter. An average serving contains probably 40 to 60 billion milliliters, so eating yogurt is an easy way to ingest many good bacteria and repopulate the gut. This is essential for people with DS because having a properly functioning GI system will, by itself, relieve much of the distress they experience.

As the probiotics grow, they consume some of the food and also produce compounds (in addition to enzymes) that help ensure good health. For instance, the colon bacteria called *Bifidobacterium* will produce butyrate, and butyrate, it turns out, is the most important food source for the cells that line the colon, the *colonocytes*. These colon cells do a number of things, assisting in the absorption of materials and in moving them from the anus. Anyone who has gone more than a couple of days without having a bowel movement can explain how important this is to general health!

To help remedy pancreatic insufficiency, taking a mixture of probiotics is recommended, as not all *Lactobacilli* are created equal, even though they are similar. The bonus of taking very high dosages is getting a lot of different enzymes that are *produced* by the probiotics, since not all of the probiotics will produce the same enzymes and at the same levels. You could get anywhere from 40 billion to several 100 billion.

What's more, the cells don't even need to be alive if all you're worried about is getting the enzymes. That's not to say you should go out and look for dead organisms or ones that are produced poorly (and some are) but rather that you don't need to incur a huge expense just to get the enzymes. Even at rest, probiotics can supply large amounts of enzymes. Most of the enzymes that probiotics make are kept inside the cells, and when the cells die, the enzymes are released. It doesn't matter *how* the cells die; the enzymes will still be released. Until the GI tract has been repaired, supplementing with large does should probably be continued.

Many people with Down syndrome have a problem with the duodenum; namely, it seems either to be closed or, in many instances, completely absent. When someone with DS has this condition, called *duodenal atresia*, large does of *Lactobacillus acidophilus* or *Lactobacillus rhamnosus* can be used for treatment. Both have great clinical data behind them and are known to be very hardy organisms.

Probiotics have been used extensively to treat celiac disease, also common among people with DS. One of the treatments for this disease is *Glucosamine HCl (GHCl)*, one of the few *prebiotics* (something able to feed probiotics) that's actually *bifidogenic*, which means it promotes the growth of *bifidobacteria* (something very few compounds can do selectively.) *Bifidobacteria* are the primary residents of the colon, and without them, we would all suffer massive infections. *Bifidobacteria* are the first probiotics to populate the GI of the infant, and as such, they set up the first line of defense for our young. Of special interest is the fact that *GHCl* is the bifidogenic material in mother's milk. The body doesn't do anything without a purpose, so it's likely that *GHCl* is there because it's important to the developing baby. In fact, *GHCl* stimulates the growth of *bifidobacterium* in the colon of the fetus.

Someone who has an enlarged colon should consume large doses of *Bifidobacterium* because these are the organisms normally found in the colon. Again, the recommendation is to start with one type of organism, add one or two more, and then rotate them. Clinically, after the initial pulse of probiotics to assist with the problem, it seems to help to rotate the organisms. Such pulsing and rotating seems to be gaining in acceptance and will soon be the norm for probiotic usage.

The success of probiotics in treating the conditions associated with Down syndrome supports the notion that there is some relationship between what's happening in the gut and in the brain. Again, neurological development seems inseparable from GI maturation. In the near future, probiotics will likely be intimately associated with all types of therapy for people with Down syndrome. The emergence of high-quality, well-researched strains will set the stage for the application of more specific pharmaceuticals.

Indeed, the future looks bright in terms of using probiotics to treat the conditions related to Down syndrome. And success in this area can only support the efforts of people with Down syndrome to lead happy, healthy, and productive lives. If nothing else, relieving some of the anxiety and misunderstanding that affects people with DS will help bring them the dignity and respect they deserve as human beings.

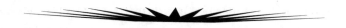

CHAPTER 10

Choosing the Best
Probiotic Delivery Systems

"It's all in the delivery!" This statement holds true for many things in life, and it can be applied to the use of probiotics, as well. Given what we've learned about the beneficial health effects of probiotics, we now have a strong ally in the war against disease and infection. All that's needed is to change the public perception regarding bacteria, reassuring them that probiotics are *good* bacteria and thus *good* for their health.

In this final chapter, I'm going to discuss some of the most interesting probiotics I have found. Also, when appropriate, I will include some data to support the theory behind the system as well as some comments from the people who developed the system. Certainly, there are other products on the market, and new ones are being developed all the time. But at present, these are the ones I think have the best science behind them. I'm not being paid by any of these companies, nor is my purpose to say anything damaging about anyone. Some of the companies are competitive with one another, however, so I have tried to include as much appropriate information as possible.

It may not seem obvious at first, but there are actually many, many different ways to take probiotics. All of these methods are basically variations on the same theme of delivering the organisms to the gastrointestinal (GI) tract. In the last 10 years, probiotic delivery systems have moved beyond the comparatively simple method of eating yogurt to include much more complicated methods, such as microencapsulation. Each method has its own advantages and disadvantages along with relevant applications.

THE TRADITIONAL
PROBIOTIC DELIVERY SYSTEM

As just mentioned, probiotics have traditionally been delivered into the body by consuming fermented dairy products, such as yogurt. There are generally two types of yogurt: homemade and storebought.

The traditional way that yogurt is made in the home involves taking some milk and either adding a starter culture to it or just letting it sit on the counter at room temperature for several days until it hardens. Both methods work well, but using a starter culture can expedite the process and plant large numbers of probiotics in the milk. In doing so, you can control what organisms go into the mix.

Typically, a starter contains at least two organisms: *Lactobacillus bulgaricus* and *Streptococcus thermophilus*. These are both great probiotics, with lots of clinical documentation and known efficacy for treating a variety of the conditions covered in this book. Other organisms that are often found in starters are *Lactobacillus acidophilus* and *Bifidobacterium bifidum*. Again, both are wonderful probiotics and should be consumed regularly.

With the latter homemade method, in which the milk is allowed to ferment on its own, you are relying on the fact that lactic acid bacteria are everywhere and will find their way into the milk. Of course, the danger here is that a lot of *other* organisms might also find their way into the milk and grow in this medium. Then, once the yogurt has formed, you won't be sure whether it's safe to eat or not.

Well, there are some clues that will give it away if the yogurt contains bad organisms. Usually, if yogurt has any real smell, it has a very pleasant dairy smell; you should look for that. If the yogurt contains bad organisms, it might be tangy and have an offensive odor, or it may form multiple layers of different consistencies or show discoloration in some part. These are some of the more obvious warning signs that indicate you should start over!

The second type of yogurt is that which is made commercially and bought in the store. Again, these yogurts almost always start with *Lactobacillus bulgaricus* and *Streptococcus thermophilus*. The organisms *Lactobacillus acidophilus* and *Bifidobacterium bifidum* are added later. Many products contain other organisms, as well, each positioned according to how the product will be marketed. For instance, if the manufacturer wants to say that they support developing a healthy immune system, they may add *Lactobacillus plantarum*, *Lactobacillus reuteri*, and/or *Lactobacillus rhamnosus*, each of which has some clinical documentation for increasing certain immune parameters thought to be desirable.

The problem with supplying probiotics through ingesting a yogurt is that the probiotics will die very quickly if there is a lot of moisture around. In fact, within one month, almost *all* the probiotics will be dead in a yogurt, even if it's kept refrigerated. That's why when you buy yogurt at the store, you should look for the expiration date. As you rummage through the dairy case, pick the container furthest back because it was likely made and delivered most recently.

Also look for a label on the container that says something like "Contains live cultures." Sometimes, you'll find a label that says "Contains live cultures at the time of manufacture." The problem is that this tells you nothing about what state the probiotics are in right *then*— when you want to purchase the product. The yogurt may even have been pasteurized, which by definition will kill the probiotics. So, review the packaging carefully to find out just what you're getting.

ALTERNATE PROBIOTIC DELIVERY SYSTEMS

Why even bother with yogurt, given these problems? Actually, you don't need to. I happen to like yogurt, so I use it. And in fact, if yogurt is prepared correctly, the number of probiotics in it can reach 100s of billions per gram, which makes it a comparatively inexpensive way of getting a lot of probiotics into the body.

However, for those of you who just don't have the time to mess around with yogurt and would rather not guess how long it's been on the shelf at a store, a variety of supplements are available that use different strategies for delivering probiotics in a viable and healthy state. I'm going to discuss these products in a later section on manufacturers. (Also see the Resources section at the end of the book for information on contacting the manufacturers and finding out about their products.)

I also urge you to talk to your doctor about the use of probiotics, just as you should about any other health concern. But I'll forewarn you: Many M.D.s are not well versed in this area. You might have better luck with an N.D. (Doctor of Naturopathy), which is what I am. Whatever the case, just make sure you find someone you are comfortable with.

Prebiotics

Before I launch into the discussion of probiotic delivery systems, I want to say a few things about prebiotics because they add to the value of a delivery system. The most common types of *prebiotics* are *Fructose oligosaccharide (FOS)* and *Inulin*. (The latter is just a really long form of the former.) FOS is simply a glucose molecule that has one or more fructose molecules attached in sequence.

One of the best prebiotics—*Glucosamine hydrochloride (GHCl)*—is not often used as such, oddly enough. You may have heard of glucosamine in the context of treating osteoarthritis; in fact, it's the basic "building block" for the cartilage in the body. Glucosamine is also the compound naturally present in mother's milk that helps protect the baby from microorganisms after birth. It does this by encouraging the growth of *Bidifobacterium*, which are extremely important in preventing infections early in life. As the baby feeds, he or she ingests this prebiotic *(GHCl)*, which supports the healthy growth and functioning of the intestines, in particular, and the baby, in general.

I have only come across one product that uses the prebiotic *GHCl* in its probiotic, and it's made by Country Life. This is one of those products that I consider brilliant in formulation because the scientists who created it had the foresight to take care of the nutrition of the probiotics as well as the human. (See Country Life in the section on manufacturers/products.)

The Brudnak Method of Pulsing and Rotating

Before learning about manufacturers and their products, there's one more important topic you should know about: the *Brudnak method* of pulsing and rotating. As noted elsewhere in this book, the Brudnak method is the current state-of-the-art technology in the use of probiotics. In it, a variety of probiotics are introduced and then substituted over the course of treatment. Most probiotics have similar effects, so people often select and use a single probiotic. But anecdotal evidence has shown that when someone supplements only with, say, *Lactobacillus acidophilus*, his or her body somehow becomes accustomed to this organism, such that it has less and less of a positive effect over time. The body seems to react differently to freshly supplied organisms, even if they are normal inhabitants of the GI.

In the *Brudnak method*, a high dose of a single strain or a limited number of strains is ingested for the initial approach—the "pulse." This dose is ingested on a regular basis for a period of time: in most cases, several days if it's a high-dose and several weeks if it's a lower dose. After that time, the body will have become accustomed to the initial treatment, so the products must be "rotated." Another dose of another strain or a mixed culture of several strains is used during this two-week phase. Finally, there is a "maintenance" dose, which should be taken over a longer period of time—daily or every other day to get the best response. This final stage is necessary because over time, probiotics undergo what is known as *genetic drift*. Put simply, they slowly mutate, ultimately to the point of dying. By taking fresh ones everyday, you can replace those that have mutated and are sick or dying. Out with the old and in with the new! That is absolutely crucial to using probiotics successfully.

If and when this series of treatments has diminishing returns, another series can be initiated using different doses and strains. The key is to stay in tune with the body, recognizing when it has become accustomed to a certain organism and then switching to something new.

How well does the Brudnak method work? Let me share the opinion of Dr. Stephanie G. Hoener, a naturopathic physician based in Portland, Oregon (see Resources for contact information), who specializes in assisting children with special needs, such as autism. She passed along the following clinical observation based on her work with these children:

> In children with autism, it is extremely common to see that they do very well on a probiotic supplement for a period of time and then it appears to lose its efficacy. For example, after starting a probiotic, they may have a resolution of their diarrhea, more well-formed stools, less gassiness and abdominal bloating, and less abdominal discomfort. If these benefits appear to lessen after a period of several weeks, we can switch them to a different strain of probiotic and the positive improvements will generally return. I've spoken with dozens of parents who have tried this pulsing-and-rotating approach with their autistic child and obtained very favorable results.

As far as I know, Pilsung Probiotics is the only manufacturer that currently uses the Brudnak method in developing its products—and they do so quite well! (See the information about Pilsung in the following section.) Other manufacturers are gradually working the Brudnak method into their existing product lines, and I've made note of this in the reviews that follow. This may take some time, but it is, indeed, happening.

Probiotic Manufacturers and Products

The products and manufacturers I discuss in this section are some of my favorites. Even so, I try not to recommend any line over another but rather to give you my impression of the science these companies are doing. In the interest of fairness, the manufacturers are organized alphabetically by company name, and specific products are identified within each manufacturer.

If you are aware of other products or things about these products that I've failed to mention, please be sure to contact me and I'll make sure your information is considered in preparing the next edition of this book.

AdvoCare

Probiotic Sachets (or Biotic Buddies). A clever system with wonderful stability is the probiotic sachet, which contains one, two, or more organisms in a tiny little packet that's not much bigger than the packet of sugar you would get at a restaurant.

The best thing I can say about this product is "Wow!" I have seen and tasted a few other sachet products, but this one is by far the best. Typically, the sachet contains a prebiotic (such as FOS) and has a creamy vanilla or orange Dreamsicle-type flavor. Everyone loves these, including kids. In fact, this improved taste is a major breakthrough because probiotics are notoriously bitter and taste like rancid milk, to be frank. The attractive pink packaging also adds to this product's "kid appeal."

The other primary selling point of the sachet is its stability, which is ideal. The shelf-life is well over a year and even close to 2 years, according to the most recent data. This is accomplished principally by using MAKTech strains, by strictly controlling the manufacturing process, and by using a multilayer sachet to keep the moisture out.

Another potential benefit of these sachet products is that they may help prevent cavities. There is mounting evidence that eating probiotics may inhibit the organisms that cause dental disease (including cavities). This is exciting news! I've heard rumors that a mouthwash is being developed that uses probiotics as part of an overall oral health program.

Dr. Richard Scheckenbach, president of R-squared Nutrition, Inc., whose background includes the rigorous program in microbiology/biochemistry at Oregon State, had this to say about AdvoCare's sachet product:

Convenience equals compliance, and there is no more

convenient way to carry or to consume highly beneficial quantities of probiotics than with AdvoCare's Biotic Buddies sachets. That combined with great taste and a pleasing mouthfeel makes daily intake (compliance) as easy for kids as for adults.

AdvoCare as a company has similarly positive things to say about Scheckenbach:

With painstaking and uncompromising care, Scheckenbach develops the formulas that set AdvoCare products apart.

I have to agree. I have worked with him on projects before and can personally attest to his professionalism and knowledge, not just about AdvoCare's products but about human biology, nutrition, and science in general.

Alticor (formerly Amway/Nutrilite)/ Access Business Group (ABG)

Intestiflora. I really like the concept used by ABG, a division of Alticor, which uses a "pixie stick" to deliver their probiotic supplement, Intestiflora. These candy-like sticks have a slightly sweet taste and are very handy, so I'm sure kids will like them, too.

An Intestiflora stick consists of 1 billion total organisms, which are divided equally between *Lactobacillus acidophilus* and *Bifidobacterium longum*—two of the most popular and asked for probiotics. For its prebiotic and carrier, this product uses the short-chained *Fructooligosaccharides* (or *scFOS*), which is sweet. There is nothing exciting about the organisms themselves, as many products have these two. What is exciting, however, is the fact that the activity of the organisms is guaranteed for 18 months!

Some companies will hedge and say they guarantee the count of organisms *at the time of manufacture*. ABG's research has resulted in a delivery system that is actually stable far beyond that, which is wonderful. When I buy a probiotic, I use it within a month or two and feel pretty sure I'm getting what the label says I'm getting (although admittedly, I look for specific brands that I know I can count on). With

ABG's product, however, I would feel safe keeping it for almost 2 years!

We all grew up knowing the name Amway and the high-quality products it stood for. And while the company is now under a new name, ABG (or Alticor), the same rigorous standards are used to test and qualify their products. I know these people well enough to know that they would not make a claim like this about the viability of Intestiflora if they were not absolutely sure. You can feel very much at ease with this product.

I spoke with Dr. Frank Welch, who is a senior research scientist for ABG and played a lead role in the design of Intestiflora. Before that, he spent much of his career working for General Mills and developing their Yoplait yogurt. So clearly, his credentials in the area of probiotics are topnotch. We had a long and pleasant talk about the general subject of probiotics and about ABG's product, in particular.

In my conversation with Dr.. Welch, I asked what he felt his prebiotic/probiotic product had to offer. He said that it was important for any such product to use strains that have been clinically tested and to provide a coating and encapsulating system to protect the organisms from being destroyed by the gastric environment. He added:

We had to make absolutely sure our probiotic product was topnotch because we are known for being so good.

I agree that both ABG and Intestiflora are topnotch!

Mr. Welch has personally devoted much time to developing a vegetable-based coating system for the probiotics. He explained this as follows:

What we succeeded in doing was creating a stable powdered delivery system. We did this so that if people did not want to take the probiotic straight from the stick, they could mix it with whatever food they wanted without adversely affecting the taste. Also, by mixing with food, it affords the probiotics a second round of protection, in addition to the coating, from the harsh gastric environment.

One of the reasons companies such as ABG (Alticor) go to great lengths to create probiotic products that can be mixed with foods is that in the United States, there is a problem with the education of consumers. Namely, people don't understand that taking probiotics is good for their health, in and of itself. Nearly all Americans have been raised to believe all bacteria are bad, *especially when they are in the body!*

In Asian countries, people view probiotics as *necessary* to good health. When Asian people are under stress, they don't reach for beta-blockers and sedatives, as Westerners sometimes do; instead, Easterners often reach for something such as a pleasant-tasting probiotic. They know that stress can knock out the bacterial flora of the GI tract and, in doing so, weaken the body, causing repercussions in other areas, including such conditions as acne and eczema. Americans, in particular, are obsessed with their outward appearance but pay little attention to how they look *inside*. (For anyone who is interested, the Alticor website provides more information about these issues; see the Resources section.)

Finally, the Intestiflora product, like the probiotic sachet discussed earlier (see AdvoCare), might help fight off the organisms that cause dental disease, including cavities. Both of these products would fit nicely into a probiotic regimen of oral health care.

BioGenesis

Pro Flora Plus. Other naturopathic physicians are catching on to the concept of using high-dose probiotics in their products, including Dr. David B. Wood, vice president, chief medical officer, and co-founder of BioGenesis Nutraceuticals, Inc. BioGenesis makes a very high-potency product called Pro Flora Plus that has 3 billion of each of the following organisms: *Lactobacillus acidophilus*, *Bifidobacterium bifidum*, and *Lactobacillus rhamnosus*. This makes a total of 9 billion organisms per capsule!

This product was designed especially to support the digestive problems of people with autism. It also makes a great transition product when switching from other probiotics, and it fits perfectly with the *Brudnak method* of pulsing and rotating strains. In fact, BioGenesis is supposed to release an entire line for this purpose some time during 2003–2004.

In a conversation with Dr. Wood, he told me that as a practicing naturopathic physician and microbiologist, he has been really disappointed in the probiotic products available. So, he was very excited about developing Pro Flora Plus, about which he had this to say:

This formula is carefully researched and provides the ideal strains of bacteria for human gastrointestinal health. Numerous studies have shown the positive health benefits from the ingestion of *L. acidophilus, Bifidobacterium,* and *L. rhamnosus.* While many companies provide *acidophilus* and *bifidus* products, most are transient flora strains, which are incapable of colonizing the human intestinal tract. Few products have *L. rhamnosus,* which may be one of the most beneficial of all the *Lactobacilli.* Studies have shown that *L. rhamnosus* can actually displace bacterial pathogens such as *Clostridium difficile* from the gut wall. . . . I believe this is a breakthrough product in the probiotic arena. It certainly will have positive health benefits, and I will be using it in my own private practice.

CHR Hansen

A unique product is offered by CHR Hansen, and it's unique in that it uses an aluminum container with a moisture scavenger in the cap of the aluminum package. While CHR Hansen is a primary manufacturer and doesn't sell to the public at large, they do sell to many of the companies you may be familiar with. Ask about this product at your local health food store; I'm sure they will be able to tell you all about it. Otherwise, contact MAK Wood, Inc., who is CHR Hansen's sales agent. (For contact information, see MAK Wood in the Resources section.)

Country Life

Acidophilus with Pectin. Each capsule contains 20 million units of active *L. acidophilus* culture plus 100 milligrams of citrus pectin.

Flora Cleanse Factors. For a healthy flora, this product offers a specialized combination of chlorella with the sensational Power-Dophilus. The triple-strain, *acidophilus*-like culture of this product, when coupled with *chlorella*, creates the ideal formulation for cleansing and purification. This product is hypoallergenic.

Maxi Baby-Dophilus. This version of Power-Dophilus was developed to satisfy the delicate needs of infants and young children. It contains just the right strains of friendly bacteria to help babies through early stages of development. This product is hypoallergenic and vegetarian.

Power-Dophilus. At 4 billion organisms per gram, this special combination of three of the most potent acidophilus-like strains is 8 to 10 times more effective than other products in achieving a healthy intestinal flora. It's also milk free and hypoallergenic.

Power-Dophilus II with Glucosamine HCl. This product nourishes the intestinal mucosal tissues and supplies organisms that produce lactic acid. It, too, is milk free and hypoallergenic. (The "staying power" of this product is also remarkable: My father was involved in its formulation, and I have been taking it for years!)

Danisco Cultor

HOWARU. HOWARU is a culture of *Bifidobacterium lactis* that was created by Danisco in collaboration with scientists from Australia and New Zealand. Some research has suggested that this bacterium by itself can enhance the levels of other indigenous probiotics. In other words, HOWARU may either condition the GI tract, making it more favorable to other probiotics, or be suitable as a sort of prebiotic, which feeds the probiotics. In any event, ingesting this product seems to help improve resistance to infection by bad bacteria such as *E. coli* and other food bacteria, perhaps by enhancing the immune system. More needs to be learned, but I am certain that such a high-quality company as Danisco will soon figure it out. In addition to being topnotch themselves, they have top-level affiliations around the world.

Dr. Lars Petersen, Danisco's scientific director for research and development, is largely credited with having built the probiotic industry in the United States. He was previously at CHR Hansen, and together with MAK Wood, they revolutionized the probiotic industry. I've worked with Dr. Petersen since the 1980s, and I can speak to his credibility. In fact, when I want quality lab work done and I can't afford to waste the time involved in someone getting it wrong a few times, I go to Dr. Petersen.

Another issue that speaks to the credibility of Danisco Cultor is that they are doing what they can to make probiotics seem user friendly—more human and less technical. The name of the product HOWARU, in fact, was inspired by the Maori word for *health*. (Since this strain originated from New Zealand, it seemed appropriate to choose a name from that culture.) Global recognition of the friendly expression "How are you?" also makes the name ideal from a marketing standpoint. As summed up on the Danisco website:

Most things related to health or the workings of the body tend to be complicated, including the scientific names of probiotic strains. Consumers still tend to be confused by such terms, and that can make it difficult for them to distinguish between good strains and those that are not so good. To help make this distinction a little easier, we came up with the user-friendly HOWARU brand.

Healthy Living Naturally (HLN)

GentlyRotate. One of the most brilliant systems of protection for probiotics I have seen is that found in GentlyRotate (by HLN), which uses the MAKTech-Matrix as part of its pulse-and-rotate protocol. Specifically, a polysaccharide weave (PW) is used to naturally coat the probiotics, which are any of the high-quality strains from MAK Wood, Inc. (See also MAK Wood later in this section.) In other words, the probiotics are protected by complex sugars (that is, more than one sugar strung together) that are strung together in such a way as to make a tight weave around the probiotics. These are not the kinds of sugars we digest; in fact, they are more fibers than sugars because of how they are bound/strung together.

The way the GentlyRotate system works is that the probiotics are actually imbedded in the PW and then encapsulated. When a capsule of this product is ingested, it goes to the stomach. There, the water naturally present in the stomach (as part of the hydrochloric acid) enters the capsule and mixes with the PW. The PW swells up and forms a gel, much like some fiber supplements do. Everything inside the gel is protected from the acid in the stomach and later the bile, as well. Only the very small outer layer of probiotics is killed off. In effect, they sacrifice themselves in order to protect their fellow bacteria inside. I have seen pictures of capsules of this product that have sat in acid for long periods of time (hours), and when they were later cracked open, the insides were completely dry! When the swollen capsule passes from the stomach to the small intestine, it dissolves because the pH of the intestine is higher than that of the stomach. The probiotics are then released intact into the intestine.

GentlyRotate is a very advanced system, and the stability data about it are wonderful—in fact, some of the best I have seen in the industry. The products in this line could be stable at room temperature for over 2 years, which is amazing. GentlyRotate is an ideal product to take with you traveling (especially if you go out of the country) because no special handling is required. I always keep a bottle with me when I am traveling.

Professional GI Line. HLN uses GentlyRotate in their Professional GI Line, which also includes the products PerfectContours and EnteroHealthy. All three are designed to fit the *Brudnak method* of pulsing and rotating probiotics. Because most of the larger manufacturers do not sell directly to everyday people, such as you and me, companies such as HLN bring their products to market. They have qualified ingredients (that is, probiotics) from Danisco and Rhodia and are in the process of qualifying CHR Hansen for use. (In Europe, they are known as *Christian Hansen's*.) Check HLN's website for updates in this area (see the Resources section).

See also entries for Danisco and Rhodia in this section.

Jarrow Formulas

Dophilus EPS Yet another interesting way of delivering probiotics is the *enteric-coated protection system (EPS)* used by Jarrow Formulas. Each capsule of Dophilus EPS is individually enteric coated and has its own blister-sealed chamber, which means the organisms it contains will be protected from saliva, stomach acid, and other digestive secretions. Extraneous sources of moisture and oxygen are excluded, as well. Because of the special coating, this product bypasses the acid barrier and delivers 4.4 billion live organisms per capsule. In short, it provides superior results with fewer capsules.

Jarrow Formulas has selected some of the most important organisms that naturally inhabit the human GI tract for inclusion in its formula. All of these are designed to stimulate the immune system and protect against intestinal pathogens. Eight different species are employed, spanning four different genera of bacteria: *Lactobacillus, Bifidobacteria, Lactococcus,* and *Pediococcus.* In addition, a flanking product (which complements the probiotic product) that uses fermented soy protein is used as the protein source.

The combination of superior starting materials, enteric coating, and individually sealed chambers means that Dophilus EPS is stable at normal room temperature. Jarrow recommends storing the product under refrigeration (and so do I), but that's an added safeguard. In sum, the entire system makes a lot of sense.

Jarrow has two of the industry's top formulators: Sid Shastri and Dr. Dallas Clouatre. Dr. Clouatre—author of *The Prostate Miracle, Anti-Fat Nutrients,* and numerous other books—had this to say about probiotics:

> The gastrointestinal tract is the gateway for the entry of all substances into the body, other than injected compounds or items brought in via the lungs. For this reason, probiotics and other supplements which directly influence the health of the GI tract can exert a powerful influence on the long-term status of the entire body. The uptake of nutrients is heavily influenced by the microbial population of the gut, and this influence extends to the absorption of minerals, such as calcium, that we

do not normally realize is dependent upon the actions of probiotics. Moreover, the microflora play a significant role in the maintenance of intestinal immune homeostasis in the prevention of inflammation, and in regulating the overall immune balance of the body.

There are so many good things to say about these products that I could write a book on the Jarrow formulas alone!

MAK Wood, Inc.

MAK Ferma Soy. Similar to the product MAK Ferma, MAK Ferma Soy has gone through one more major step: The probiotics have been grown in the presence of soy protein, which they ferment, or utilize as a food source. The reason for doing this is that one of the enzymes that probiotics make in this process is very unique. That enzyme, *alpha-glucosidase*, takes the unabsorbable (or of very low solubility) form of isoflavones (which are natural products that act like estrogen) and cuts off the sugar molecules attached. After that happens, the isoflavones are much more absorbable and hence much more functional in the body. The MAK Ferma concept is absolutely brilliant, something that companies such as Jarrow recognize and use in creating their own products.

MAKTech. Recently, MAK Wood formalized how they create a probiotic product using a process called MAKTech. In short, it's a scientific validation program to ensure that the products are of the highest quality possible. Each product is backed by scientific validation in the published literature. If there is no science behind a product, the company will not sell it.

In particular, the MAKTech probiotics pass a rigorous series of tests, which may include DNA fingerprinting, DNA agarose (a highly purified agur) gel electrophoresis, cell-surface carbohydrate structure determination, and biochemical analysis of the probiotic strains. This is all state of the art in terms of the available science in this area.

The whole MAKTech process follows all the ingredients from the country of origin to the final product, which has to be approved before shipping.

MAKTech-Matrix. This is one of the most brilliant systems of protection for probiotics I have seen. Specifically, a polysaccharide weave (PW) is used to naturally coat the probiotics, which are any of the high-quality strains from MAK Wood, Inc. In other words, the probiotics are protected by complex sugars (that is, more than one sugar strung together) that are strung together in such a way as to make a tight weave around the probiotics. These are not the kinds of sugars we digest; in fact, they are more fibers than sugars because of how they are bound/strung together.

For more on this system, see the section on Healthy Living Naturally (HLN). HLN's product GentlyRotate uses the MAKTech-Matrix.

Matol Botanical International

Fibresonic. An interesting probiotic delivery vehicle is manufactured by a Canadian company, Matol. They have a product called Fibresonic, which is high in fiber (both soluble and insoluble), low in fat and cholesterol, and rich in healthy nutrients and essential vitamins and minerals. The high level of fiber in this product is particularly noteworthy, as fiber is known for its ability to combat both high cholesterol levels and intestinal diseases such as colon cancer, diverticulitis, and chronic constipation.

A review of the list of ingredients reveals that Fibresonic also contains the probiotic *Lactobacillus acidophilus* (although Matol doesn't promote this fact). Fiber and probiotics—what a fantastic combination! The fiber works like a scrub brush, cleaning out the old, dead material, and the probiotics help boost the bacterial population. Everyone can benefit from Fibresonic's good-tasting and easy-to-use fiber delivery system.

Beta Glucan Product. Matol also has another product with beta glucan, which is a wonderful compliment to probiotics. The beta glucans were provided by a high-quality supplier.

Enzymes with Probiotics. I have written extensively on the topic of using enzymes with probiotics for various applications, so I was thrilled when I saw this product. It not only contains high-quality enzymes but also the following blend of probiotics: *Bifidobacterium bifidum, Lactobacillus brevis, Bifidobacterium longum, Lactobacillus acidophilus,* and *Lactobacillus rhamnosus.*

This is a wonderful product, and I can see it only improving as the strains and enzymes are further refined. This product would fit well with the *Brudnak method* of pulsing and rotating probiotics. Specifically, it would make a great transition product when switching from one "pulse" of high-dose probiotics to another high dose of a single or a few probiotics. I would also recommend this product as a "maintenance" product for use in keeping the usual endogenous probiotics in your body at normal levels.

In the brochure for this product, Georges Morisset, Ph.D., of Matol, said:

> I have become much more aware of the importance of enzymes on our health since I joined Matol. My personal research has easily convinced me of the key role they play in the absorption of our foods so we can fully metabolize all the nutrients we eat. They are not called "the sparks of life" for nothing. They assist in practically all bodily functions and we all know many of the enzymes in our foods are destroyed by the way we cook and the way they are processed.

Natren

Trenev Trio. Another of my favorites is a product from Natren called the Trenev Trio, which contains *Lactobacillus acidophilus* (NAS superstrain), *Bifidobacterium bifidum* (Malyoth superstrain), and *Lactobacillus bulgaricus* (LB-51 superstrain) all in one capsule. Natren's probiotic supplements are uniquely distinguished from other products because of the selection of certain superstrains and the efficacious delivery systems, which are designed to maximize survival and growth in the intestines.

The Trenev Trio is one of the most interesting products on the market. In addition to the three strains of probiotics mentioned, one capsule also contains sunflower oil and vitamin E. And finally, all of the oxygen and water have been removed from the capsule, thereby creating a totally anaerobic environment. This is important because both oxygen and water are bad for probiotics.

In their normal environment, which is the intestines, probiotics are used to living without oxygen and water (or having them in very small amounts). Oxygen can actually destroy some of the bacteria, while water supports their living. In this case, we don't want the probiotics to go about living; they will wear themselves out and have limited viability and shelf life. (This is why yogurt cultures are only good for a month or so.) We don't want the probiotics dead but rather just "asleep," or in *stasis*. Removing the water puts the probiotics in a state of suspended animation.

This revolutionary development had never been tried before, and I give a lot of credit to Natren for pioneering it. This system totally separates and protects the *acidophilus, bifidum,* and *bulgaricus* cells until they're called into action in the GI tract. The cells are literally *microenrobed*, or protected from the onslaught of gastric juices and each other. In vitro tests of the Trenev Trio showed that the organisms protected by the oil matrix survived 1 hour in a simulated gastric juice environment to which trypsin and pepsin had been added. (These are very strong enzymes that can digest proteins in other bacteria and kill them.) Other in vitro studies have shown that this product may be capable of the following:

- Producing bactericidal metabolites, including hydrogen peroxide
- Suppressing the adherence or growth of pathogenic bacteria and reducing their ability to colonize the GI tract
- Inhibiting the translocation of pathogenic bacteria across the intestinal wall and thereby preventing infections
- Enhancing the degradation of toxins produced by pathogenic bacteria
- Enhancing the production of antibodies and stimulating the

production of phyagocytes (that is, white blood cells essential for proper functioning of the immune system)

- Assimilating cholesterol
- Releasing lactase, the enzyme responsible for the digestion of milk lactose
- Producing strong organic acids that inhibit the growth of undesirable pathogenic organisms
- Suppressing harmful bacteria that may ultimately lead to aging and the development of geriatric diseases
- Lowering the fecal pH, which in turn decreases the ammonia level
- Increasing the body's absorption of nutrients such as calcium, which is important for postmenopausal women

I asked Dr. Natasha Trenev, the owner of Natren, where she saw probiotics going in the future, and she said that strain identification is "going to be one of the most important issues in the years to come." I completely agree with her on this. Strain identification will be vital in preventing would-be companies from falsely claiming that they are selling expensive strains, when their products don't really contain those strains at all.

Natasha's Probiotic Face Cream. Natren also has a unique product called Natasha's Probiotic Face Cream, and again, I believe the idea behind it is sound. Probiotics are not just in the body; they are also *on* the body. Likewise, there are bad bacteria on the surface of the body, especially the face, and they can either cause or worsen a number of conditions, such as acne. Applying Natren's face cream should help prevent the growth of these bad bacteria and help control these conditions. This just seems like one of those products that makes sense.

Nature's Sunshine

This company makes only a few probiotic products, but what they do make is stellar. I know a lot of naturopaths who use these products.

Bifidophilus Flora Force. This product contains 2.5 billion *acidophilus* and 1 billion *Bifidobacterium longum* per capsule, for a total of 3.5 billion microorganisms per capsule. Each capsule also contains 100 milligrams of *fructooligosaccharide* (dietary fiber) plus carrot powder to provide nourishment for the bacteria. The cultures are freeze dried to preserve their viability, and the product should be refrigerated or frozen to maintain freshness. This product contains no milk, wheat, or soy products and no preservatives.

Flora Force (L. Acidophilus). Designed for anyone who wants a large count of *L. acidophilus* in one capsule, this product yields a minimum of 2 billion bacteria per capsule to help repopulate the intestinal tract. The *L. acidophilus* is cultured in carrot juice before being freeze dried, and each capsule is enterically coated to ensure that the culture will be released only in the intestinal tract. This product contains no milk, wheat, corn, or soy products.

Nature's Way

Over the years, Nature's Way has developed the following products with an enormous amount of support (that is, purchases) from people like you and me. In fact, my whole family takes these products.

Nature's Way Primadophilus Bifidus. This product, which is intended primarily for those over 50 years of age, contains 10 billion microorganisms per gram (at the time of manufacture) of specially selected strains *Bifidobacterium* and *Lactobacillus*. This product is freeze dried.

Nature's Way Primadophilus for Children. This is an easy-to-use powder that mixes quickly with any liquid, infant formula, or food. There is a minimum potency of 1 billion *Bifidobacterium* and *Lactobacillus microorganisms* (at the time of manufacture) per one-half level teaspoon of powder.

Nature's Way Primadophilus Junior. This product is a small, easy-to-swallow, enteric-coated capsule that contains a minimum potency of 5.2 billion *Bifidobacterium* and *Lactobacillus* microorganisms per gram (at the time of manufacture).

NOW Foods

Stabilized Acidophilus. This is a company that knows their probiotics and their products! For instance, they have Stabilized Acidophilus, a real-time, lab-tested acidophilus. Because some strains of acidophilus are more stable then others, scientists have developed a proprietary method that optimizes the growth medium during fermentation. This method uses specific fermentation and drying techniques to ensure that each batch of stabilized acidophilus contains the hardiest strains of this important probiotic. In addition, substantial overages are incorporated to guarantee full potency at room temperature for the entire life of the product. Finally, stabilized acidophilus is packaged in glass for maximum protection from moisture.

4X6 Acidophilus Powder. This balanced blend of microorganisms will remain relatively stable when refrigerated. The product 4X6 Acidophilus-Dairy Free-Refrigerate has been improved to provide higher potencies and a more balanced spectrum of beneficial bacteria found in human intestinal tracts. Regular intake of beneficial probiotics can aid in maintaining healthy intestinal flora.

The label reads as follows:

Amount Per Serving		% Daily Value
14 Billion organisms per gram at time of manufacture		
Lactobacillus acidophilus	2 Billion	50%
Bifidobacterium bifidum	1.2 Billion	30%
Bifidobacterium longum	200 Million	5%
Streptococcus thermophilus	200 Million	5%
Lactobacillus bulgaricus	200 Million	5%
Lactobacillus paracasei	200 Million	5%

* Percent Daily Values are based on 2,000 calorie diet.

† Daily Value not established.

They also have an 8 billion acidophilus & bifidus blend with a label that reads:

Servings Per Container: 60

Amount Per Serving		% Daily Value
Lactobacillus acidophilus	4.0 Billion	50%
Bifidobacterium lactis	3.2 Billion	40%
Bifidobacterium longum	0.8 Billion	10%
Total minimum microorganisms	8.0 Billion	100%

What should be immediately apparent is that these all fit in nicely with the *Brudnak method* of pulsing and rotating probiotics! They are a perfect combination.

GR-8 Dophilus. Continuing with that, they also have the GR-8 Dophilus – 8 Strains 4 Billion Potency product. This one is nice because it adds in rhamnosus. The label reads:

Amount Per Serving	% Daily Value
Lactobacillus rhamnosus (Rosell-11)	600 million*
Lactobacillus acidophilus (Rosell-52)	1.2 billion*
Blend of 8 Strains of Probiotic Bacteria	4.0 Billion Organisms*
Lactobacillus casei (Rosell-215)	600 million*
Lactobacillus rhamnosus (Rosell-49)	600 million*
Bifidobacterium longum (Rosell-175)	200 million*
Pediococcus acidilactici (Rosell-1)	200 million*

If you are looking for pulsing and rotating of the strains, NOW Foods is the place to be. I personally know the director of their quality assurance department, Dr. James Roza and know he stands for what he believes in. Their unique blends of probiotic strains, coupled with their commitment to quality assurance, helps make them stand out.

Pilsung Probiotics

First of all, let me say that I love this name! *Pilsung* means "Faith in Certain Victory" in Korean, which is perfect for our purpose of fighting the war against pathogenic bacteria and disease. Pilsung is one of the leading companies that's delivering probiotics in a new way: by using a large number of them and basically overwhelming the pathogenic organisms along with the harsh gastric environment. Pilsung is also using a special methodology in the area of treating autism and associated developmental conditions. They have designed not just one or two probiotic products but an entire line that employs very high numbers of organisms.

As mentioned earlier, I believe Pilsung Probiotics is the only company currently using the state-of-the-art technology of the *Brudnak method* of pulsing and rotating in its entire line. In applying this method, Pilsung has used a high dose of a single strain or a limited number of strains for the initial approach—the "pulse." For instance, for a quick and effective way to treat diarrhea, they have a product that contains *L. rhamnosus* (30 billion organisms per dose). This is often sufficient for an isolated case of diarrhea, but for many other conditions, such as autism, diarrhea can be chronic and require constant support. After a few weeks, when the body has become accustomed to the initial *L. rhamnosus* treatment, the products are "rotated" and something else is used, such as a mixed culture of *Lactobacillus*. Then after that, a mixed culture of *Lactobacillus* and *Bifidobacterium* is taken. After that, a mixed culture of the two is ingested. Finally, there is the "maintenance" dose, which should be taken over a longer period of time.

If and when this series of treatments has diminishing returns, Pilsung Probiotics has another product that uses completely different organisms that have only recently become available: *Lactobacillus plantarum* and *Lactobacillus salivarius*. And what's really interesting about this product is that it combines these organisms with *beta glucan*, a normal component of the yeast cell wall. This is what's responsible for the product's recognition by the immune system. When beta glucan is ingested, it makes the body think there is an infection with a microorganism because only microorganisms contain this particular beta glucan. In addition, when the body thinks it's under assault, it "revs up" its immune defenses. In effect, the immune system is enhanced not just from the probiotics but also from the beta glucan.

This entire delivery system offers many advantages, including flexibility in both the dosing and the organisms used. Also, the products are packaged under nitrogen gas, which has the beneficial effect of removing oxygen and moisture, both of which are bad for probiotics (as discussed earlier).

Rhodia

Another company that's helping to advance the probioitics market is the French company Rhodia, one of the world's leading manufacturers of specialty chemicals. It provides a wide range of innovative products and services to the automotive, food, health care, cosmetics, apparel, and environmental markets by offering its customers tailor-made solutions based on the cross-fertilization of its technologies and markets. Rhodia entered the area of probiotics in the early 1970s by introducing the highly documented *Lactobacillus acidophilus* NCFM. Since then, Rhodia has expanded its offerings to include the widest range of probiotics in the industry.

I spoke with Scott Bush, business development director for Rhodia, and he had this to say about the company's probiotics program:

The cornerstone of Rhodia's probiotic business is the principle of customer partnership. We aim to cooperate with our customers to mutually achieve the goal of providing consumers with safe, stable, efficacious probiotics in a variety of delivery vehicles.

Shaklee Corporation

Optiflora. One method of protecting the probiotics as they traverse the upper GI tract (which is where they have the greatest chance of being killed) is to *microencapsulate* them. And one of the companies that has pioneered this method is the Shaklee Corporation. They have patented a state-of-the-art, triple-encapsulation process that uses natural ingredients to protect the probiotics until they are released in the large and small intestines. In addition, Shaklee has tested the effectiveness of their product under different conditions—that is, having an empty stomach and having a full stomach—both of which have certain negative effects on probiotics.

When the stomach is empty, the pH is very low and thus the probiotics will be destroyed if not protected. When the stomach is full, there is an increased secretion of acid and also greater bile production and secretion. Shaklee tested the viability (or survival) of probiotics under both of these conditions and found that their product, Optiflora, had a nearly 100 percent survival rate in comparison to 0 percent to 42 percent for two competitors' products. Optiflora also includes prebiotics, which I am very much in favor of using.

As I understand it, Shaklee has two different versions of this product, both labeled with the brand name Optiflora. Both products guarantee live delivery of *bifidus* and *acidophilus* to the intestines (both large and small).

I spoke with Shaklee's product director, Anjana Srivastava, who has devoted much of her time to developing the Optiflora products. After reviewing this section about Shaklee, she said:

> You have done an excellent job in describing our product. The only thing I would like to add is that Shaklee Corporation has spent a large amount of resources developing the technology for this room temperature stable product. We have the *exclusive* rights to this product for our market, and it requires no refrigeration.

It's easy to understand why a company would want exclusivity on such a fabulous product. As I said, the technology of Optiflora is state of the art, so it's definitely worth looking at when deciding what you should buy. And given the demonstrable technical assistance that Shaklee provides at all levels (everyone is so nice!), this company is a favorite of mine.

Solaray/Nutraceutical Corporation

Solaray is one of the brand names manufactured by parent company Nutraceutical Corporation, which also sells products under the brand names KAL, NaturalMax, VegLife, Premier One, Sunny Green, Natural Sport, ActiPet, Action Labs, Ultimate Nutrition, and Thompson. In fact, an Internet search provided a huge list of products from the Nutraceutical family.

Solaray began manufacturing and selling herbal products in 1973, originally as a pioneer in formulating and marketing blended herbal products that contain two or more herbs with complementary effects. And today, they have several very interesting probiotics.

After a little investigation, what should strike you about these products are two things: First, the extreme uniqueness of these products, such as the one with carrot juice, is very difficult to achieve these days. Second, as you can see from the list that follows, the sheer number of products is amazing!

Acidophilus Plus Carrot Juice. This juice contains over 3 billion living microorganisms per capsule. It's nondairy and freeze dried.

Acidophilus Plus Goat's Milk. Each capsule of this dietary supplement contains over 3 billion viable *L. acidophilus* organisms with additional *L. bulgaricus* and *S. thermophilus* in a base of lowfat goat's milk. It's freeze dried and has megapotency.

BabyLife Products. These products include a powder and a dietary supplement: the nondairy, freeze-dried, Super Digestaway. Over 4 billion living organisms are provided per gram. Infants, small children, and expectant and nursing mothers can all enjoy these products.

CranDophilus Products. These dietary supplements, which contain important intestinal flora, are used to keep the urinary tract healthy. Specific product names are CranDophilus, CranActin, and Cranberry AFTM Extract.

Multidophilus. A single dose of this dietary supplement contains over 1 billion each of *L. bulgaricus*, *L. acidophilus*, and *bifidus* (*B. bifidum*). It's nondairy and freeze dried.

Multidophilus Lactic Flora (3 billion). This dietary supplement contains 3 billion of the following lactic flora: *L. bulgaricus, L. acidophilus,* and *bifidus* (*B. Bifidum*). This product is nondairy and freeze dried.

Multidophilus Lactic Flora (10 billion). This powdered dietary supplement contains 10 billion of the following living microorganisms in every gram: *L. bulgaricus, L. acidophilus, bifidu*s (*B. bifidum*). This product is nondairy and freeze dried; it's packed by weight, not volume.

Multidophilus Plus DDS-1. This nondairy product is a special combination of important intestinal flora: DDS1 *Lactobacillus* spp., *L. bulgaricus, L. acidophilus,* and *bifidus* (*B. bifidum*). Each capsule supplies over 4 billion (at the time of manufacture) viable microorganisms.

Multidophilus Plus DDS-1 Black Cherry Chewables. This delicious nondairy, black cherry–flavored chewable is a special combination of important intestinal flora: *DDS1 Lactobacillus* spp., *L. bulgaricus, L. acidophilus,* and *bifidus* (*B. bifidum*). Each chewable supplies over 4 billion (at the time of manufacture) viable microorganisms.

Multidophilus Plus DDS-1 Orange Cream Chewables. These delicious, nondairy, orange-flavored chewables are a special combination of important intestinal flora: *DDS1 Lactobacillus spp., L. bulgaricus, L. acidophilus,* and *bifidus* (*B. bifidum*). Each chewable supplies over 4 billion (at the time of manufacture) viable microorganisms.

ReFresh. This dietary supplement contains *Lactobacillus acidophilus* plus an aloe vera gel concentrate, an alfalfa juice concentrate, and a rosemary herbal extract. Its purpose is to cleanse, soothe, and fortify the GI tract.

Solgar Vitamin and Herb Company

The Solgar line of products is known for having high quality and using leading-edge technology, so the Brudnak method of pulsing and rotating is a natural fit for them. Solgar has a whole line of various blends that work well with this methodology. As a consultant, I have found that these products often fit nicely into the health support plans I help people develop. And I personally look for that famous gold label whenever I walk into a health food store. I am very comfortable recommending Solgar's products. In fact, if your local health food store or grocery chain doesn't carry these products, speak to the manager and ask for them specifically. They are that good!

USANA Health Sciences

Another great idea for a delivery system was recently developed by USANA Health Sciences, of Salt Lake City, Utah, which combines probiotics and enzymes into a drink. USANA has found a way around the stability issue that comes with adding water by filling the bottle just with the powdered mixture. The consumer then adds water, shakes the bottle, and *voila*! This product is still under development, but I have tasted it and it's fantastic!

I spoke with the technical staff at USANA, which includes Dr. Gale Rudolph, the author of many written project proposals for beverages and various dry mix applications of pre- and probiotics—some of them going back to 1990. In discussing the state of research on probiotics, Dr. Rudolph said:

> With more conservative companies, the concepts haven't gotten farther than some basic formulations and variations on that theme. For other companies, however, who allow ephedra and pro-hormones, the probiotics barely pique interest. They just want something that is going to "pump you up."

The struggle that companies have is with *marketing*. Many marketers don't like probiotics due to lack of understanding or because probiotics deal with the inside of the body (and no one sees that!). At USANA, Dr. Rudolph has defended under heavy scrutiny the clinical findings that are available, even though there are hundreds of them. Her feeling is that GI health is not considered relevant or important in Western culture. People don't understand probiotics and thus don't see the need for them. She went on to say:

Until this acceptability comes about, it will be difficult to get companies to market the products. Yogurt is okay because it is a food in its own right. Dietary fiber supplements are like prune juice—for old people. Not socially acceptable. Probiotics might be sexier than fiber, but [they are] still perceived as "something must be wrong with you."

This will change when people realize that probiotics may assist with living a higher-quality life and also with looking better (by losing weight, for instance)! *Then*, probiotics will be sexy!

CHOOSING A PROBIOTIC

Again, the delivery systems just discussed are some of my favorites. I think each has unique advantages that should be explored and tested by anyone interested in using probiotics. After all, you are your own best laboratory, and these products are perfectly safe.

So, what should you look for when choosing a probiotic? Foremost, look for scientific backing. Go on the Internet to the website medline.com, and see who has published what about which products. Get familiar with the names of strains commonly used, the doses of organisms found in most products, and so on. If you develop your working knowledge in this area, you will be able to make your way more efficiently through the research and literature.

Also find out about where you can buy probiotic products. Most of the major companies—such as CHR Hansen, Danisco, MAK Wood, and Rhodia—do not sell to end users, like you and me. Rather, they sell either directly to other companies (whose names we see on the products on store shelves and in catalogs), or they use a sales agent to do that. Spend some time learning about these companies and their products because they all have something to offer.

In addition to quality control, the other real benefit of all the improved technology that's being used today is that you will get better results from the products you use. As Dr. Rudolph from USANA alluded to earlier, the probiotic market has been steadily developing and is on the verge of a massive expansion in the United States. More products will be available and not only in the health food market. Probiotics will make their way *en masse* into the food-processing arena, as well.

Despite these advances, the image problem of "probiotics as bacteria" must still be overcome in order for these products to be widely accepted and used. As mentioned earlier, the company Danisco Cultor is trying to make probiotics seem user friendly, in part, by naming one of their products in personal, friendly terms. The name HOWARU was inspired by the Maori word for *health*. Plus, there's a certain global recognition of the friendly expression "How are you?" which makes the name ideal from a marketing standpoint. Given the lack of understanding by the lay public, it makes a great deal of sense to do this.

Another company that's helping to advance the probiotics market is the French company Rhodia, one of the world's leading manufacturers of specialty chemicals. This company, also described earlier, entered the area of probiotics in the early 1970s and has since expanded its product line to include the widest range of probiotics in the industry. Rhodia also has its eye on the consumer, stating the "cornerstone" of their business in "the principle of customer partnership."

It's companies like this who have been responsible for the explosion of knowledge and product development in the area of probiotics. The interest in academia has also grown in recent years from something peripheral to something more mainstream, which is very encouraging. And while sales in the natural products market have been down over the last few years, sales of probiotics have soared.

There is only one reason for all this interest and support: *Probiotics work!* I hope I have convinced you of that throughout this book and that you will join in my passion for this subject. No matter what your condition of health, probiotics can improve it.

I'm confident in saying that probiotics are the future. We will soon see a revolution in the war on disease. As new strains of organisms are identified and made available for mass consumption, our army of allies will grow and we will enjoy success in fighting disease and perhaps in

conquering death itself. As the saying goes, "Death begins in the colon."
Now you know why!

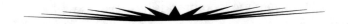

Resources

AdvoCare
2727 Realty Road
Suite 134
Carrollton, TX 75006
Phone: 972-478-4500
Fax: 972-478-4758
Web: www.advocare.com

Alticor/Access
Business Group (ABG)
Phone: 800-253-6500
Web: www.quixtar.com

Amway
See Alticor/Access
Business Group (ABG)

BioGenesis Nutraceuticals, Inc.
18303 Bothell-Everett Highway
Suite 110
Mill Creek, WA 98012
Phone: 866-272-0500
Fax: 425-485-3518
Web: www.bio-genesis.com

Brudnak, Mark A., Ph.D., N.D.
957 Lake Shore Road
Grafton, WI 53024
Phone: 414-491-4512

Cancer Information Center (CIS)
Phone: 1-800-4-CANCER

CHR Hansen, Inc.
9015 West Maple Street
Milwaukee, WI 53214
Phone: 800-558-0802
Fax: 414-607-5959
Web: www.chr-hansen.com

Country Life
180 Vanderbilt Motor Parkway
Hauppauge, NY 11788
Phone: 800-645-5768
Web: www.country-life.com

Danisco Cultor
201 New Century Parkway
New Century, KS 66031-0026
Phone: 800-255-6837
Fax: 913-764-5407
Web: www.howaru.com

Healthy Living Naturally (HLN)
Phone: 262-375-0375
Web: home.wi.rr.com/hln

Hoener, Stephanie G., N.D.
P.O. Box 155
Wilsonville, OR 97070

Jarrow Formulas, Inc.
1824 South Robertson Boulevard
Los Angeles, CA 90035
Phone: 800-726-0886
Fax: 800-890-8955
Web: www.jarrow.com

Klaire Laboratories, Inc.
140 Marine View Avenue
Suite 110
Solana Beach, CA 92075
Phone: 800-859-8358
Fax: 858-350-7883
Web: www.klaire.com

Lifeway Foods, Inc.
6431 West Oakton Avenue
Morton Grove, IL
Phone: 847-967-1010
Web: www.kefir.com

MAK Wood, Inc.
1235 Dakota Drive
Unit E
Grafton, WI 53024
Phone: 262-387-1200
Fax: 262-387-1400
Web:
home.earthlink.net/~makwood

Matol Botanical International, Ltd.
290 Labrosse Avenue
Pointe-Claire, Quebec, Canada
H9R 6R6
Phone: 800-363-6286
Fax: 800-363-8890
Web: www.matol.com

Natren, Inc.
3105 Willow Lane
Westlake Village, CA 91361
Phone: 800-992-3323
Web: www.natren.com

Nature's Sunshine Products
1655 North Main Street
Spanish Fork, UT 84660
Phone: 800-223-8225
Web: www.naturessunshine.com

Nature's Way
10 Mountain Springs Parkway
Springville, UT 84663
Phone: 801-489-1500
Fax: 801-489-1700
Web: www.naturesway.com

NOW Foods
395 South Glen Ellyn Road
Bloomingdale, IL 60108
Phone: 630-545-9098
Web: www.nowfoods.com

Nutraceutical Corporation
1400 Kearns Boulevard
Park City, UT 84060
Phone: 800-669-8877
Fax: 800-767-8514
Web: www.nutraceutical.com

Pilsung Probiotics
Phone: 414-581-5160

Rhodia
2802 Walton Commons West
Madison, WI 53718
Phone: 608-224-3117
Fax: 608-224-3186
Web: www.us.rhodia.com

Shaklee Corporation
4747 Willow Road
Pleasanton, CA 94588
Phone: 925-924-2000
Fax: 925-924-2862
Web: www.shaklee.com

Solaray
See Nutraceutical Corporation

Solgar Vitamin and Herb
Company
500 Willow Tree Road
Leonia, NJ 07605
Phone: 877-765-4274
Web: www.solgar.com

USANA Health Sciences, Inc.
3838 West Parkway Boulevard
Salt Lake City, UT 84120
Phone: 888-950-9595
Web: www.usana.com

Bibliography

Aarnikunnas J, Ronnholm K, Palva A. *The mannitol dehydrogenase gene (mdh) from Leuconostoc mesenteroides is distinct from other known bacterial mdh genes.* Appl Microbiol Biotechnol. 2002 Sep;59(6):665–71.

Adams MR. *Safety of industrial lactic acid bacteria.* J Biotechnol. 1999 Feb 19;68(2–3):171–8. Review.

Ahuja MC, Khamar B. Antibiotic associated diarrhea: *A controlled study comparing plain antibiotics with those containing protected lactobacilli.* J Indian Med Assoc. 2002 May;100(5):334–5.

Ayala-Grosso C, Ng G, Roy S, Robertson GS. *Caspase-cleaved amyloid precursor protein in Alzheimer's disease.* Brain Pathol. 2002 Oct;12(4):430–41.

Bornet FR, Brouns F. *Immune-stimulating and gut health-promoting properties of short-chain fructo-oligosaccharides.* Nutr Rev. 2002 Oct;60(10 Pt 1):326–34.

Borruel N, Carol M, Casellas F, Antolin M, De Lara F, Espin E, Naval J, Guarner F, Malagelada JR. *Increased mucosal tumour necrosis factor alpha production in Crohn's disease can be downregulated ex vivo by probiotic bacteria.* Gut. 2002 Nov;51(5):659–64.

Brudnak, MA. *Application of genomeceuticals to the molecular and immunological aspects of autism.* Med Hypotheses. 2001 May; 57(2):186–91.

Brudnak, MA. *Application of genomecuticals to the molecular and immunological aspects of autism.* ANMA The Montitor. 2001 Dec:13–22.

Brudnak MA. *Application of genomeceuticals to the molecular and immunological aspects of autism.* Presentation delivered at Nutritionals 2002 May, Anaheim, CA, 2002.

Brudnak MA. *Cancer preventing properties of essential oil Monoterpenes D-Limonene and Perillyl alcohol.* Poss Health. 2000 June;53:23–5.

Brudnak MA. *Enzyme therapy: Part II.* TLDP. 2001 Jan:94–8.

Brudnak, MA. *Genomic multi-level nutrient-sensing pathways.* Med Hypotheses. 2001 Feb;56(2):194–9.

Brudnak, MA. *High-dose probiotics for detoxification.* TLDP. 2002 Nov:110–3.

Brudnak, MA. *Nutritional regulation of gene expression.* Theory in Biosciences. 2001 March;120(1):64–75.

Brudnak, MA. *Probiotics and autism.* TLDP. 2001 April;(4):66–7.

Brudnak, MA. *Probiotics and heart disease.* The Monitor. ANMA. 2002 Aug;6(3):18–25.

Brudnak MA. *Probiotics as an adjuvant to detoxification protocols.* Med Hypotheses. 2002 May;58(5):382–5.

Brudnak MA. *Weight-loss drugs and supplements: are there safer alternatives?* Med Hypotheses. 2002 Jan;58(1):28–33.

Brudnak MA, Buchholz I, Hoener S, Newman L, Pangborn J. *Guide to intestinal health in autism spectrum disorders.* Kirkman Laboratories, 2001.

Brudnak MA, Dondero A, Van Hecke FM. *Are the "hard" martial arts, such as the Korean martial art TaeKwon-Do, of benefit to senior citizens?* Med Hypotheses. 2002 Oct;59(4):485–91.

Brudnak, MA, Hoener, SG. *Can probiotics be used for oral health?* In preparation.

Brudnak MA, Hoener SG. *Enzyme inhibitors and enzyme enhancers: Applications to autism and beyond.* In preparation.

Brudnak, MA, Miller KS. *Expression cloning exploiting PCR rescue of transfected genes.* Biotechniq. 1993 Jan;14(1):66–8.

Brudnak MA, Rimland B, Kerry RE, Dailey M, Taylor R, Stayton B, Waickman F, Waickman M, Pangborn J, Buchholz I. *Beneficial effects of enzyme-based therapy for autism. In preparation.*

Brudnak MA, Rimland B, Kerry RE, Dailey M, Taylor R, Stayton B, Waickman F, Waickman M, Pangborn J, Buchholz I. *Enzyme-based therapy for autism spectrum disorders—Is it worth another look?* Med Hypotheses. 2002 May;58(5):422–8.

Cerrato PL. *Can "healthy" bacteria ward off disease?* RN. 2000 April;63(4):71–4. Review.

Clouatre D. *Anti-fat nutrients*, 4th ed. Basic Media, 2003.

Clouatre D. *The prostate miracle*. Kensington, 2000.

Delia P, Sansotta G, Donato V, Messina G, Frosina P, Pergolizzi S, De Renzis C, Famularo G. *Prevention of radiation-induced diarrhea with the use of VSL#3, a new high-potency probiotic preparation.* Am J Gastroenterol. 2002 Aug;97(8):2150–2.

Eizaguirre I, Urkia NG, Asensio AB, Zubillaga I, Zubillaga P, Vidales C, Garcia-Arenzana JM, Aldazabal P. *Probiotic supplementation reduces the risk of bacterial translocation in experimental short bowel syndrome.* J Pediatr Surg. 2002 May;37(5):699–702.

Evans JS, Huffman S. *Update on medications used to treat gastrointestinal disease in children.* Curr Opin Pediatr. 1999 Oct;11(5):396–401. Review

Femia AP, Luceri C, Dolara P, Giannini A, Biggeri A, Salvadori M, Clune Y, Collins KJ, Paglierani M, Caderni G. *Antitumorigenic activity of the prebiotic inulin enriched with oligofructose in combination with the* probiotics *Lactobacillus rhamnosus* and *Bifidobacterium lactis* on *azoxymethane-induced colon carcinogenesis in rats.* Carcinogenesis. 2002 Nov;23(11):1953–60.

Fric P. *Probiotics in gastroenterology.* Z Gastroenterol. 2002 Mar;40(3):197–201. Review.

Gill HS, Rutherfurd KJ, Cross ML. *Dietary probiotic supplementation enhances natural killer cell activity in the elderly: an investigation of age-related immunological changes.* J Clin Immunol. 2001 Jul;21(4):264–71.

Gilliland SE, Walker DK. *Factors to consider when selecting a culture of Lactobacillus acidophilus as a dietary adjunct to produce a hypocholesterolemic effect in humans.* J Dairy Sci. 1990;73:905–911.

Gotz VP, Romankiewicz C, Moss JA, Murray HW. *Prophylaxis against ampicillin-associated diarrhea with a Lactobacillus preparation.* Am J Hosp Pharm. 1979;36:754–7.

Guetmonde M, Nieves C, Vinderola G, Reinheimer J, de los Reyes-Gavilan CG. *Evolution of carbohydrate fraction in carbonated fermented milks as affected by beta-galactosidase activity of starter strains.* J Dairy Res. 2002 Feb;69(1):125–37.

Hallen A, Jarstrand C, Pahlson C. Treatment of bacterial vaginosis with Lactobacilli. *Sexually transmitted diseases.* Nutr Clin Care. 1992 May–June;5(1):3–8. Review.

Hasler CM.Pre- and probiotics: *Where are we today?* Introduction. Br J Nutr. 1998 Oct;80(4):S195.

Heyman M, Menard S. *Probiotic microorganisms: how they affect intestinal pathophysiology.* Cell Mol Life Sci. 2002 Jul;59(7):1151–65. Review

Ishibashi N, Yamazaki S. *Probiotics and safety.* Am J Clin Nutr. 2001 Feb;73(2 Suppl):465S–70S. Review.

Johnson IT. *New food components and gastrointestinal health.* Proc Nutr Soc. 2001 Nov;60(4):481–8. Review.

Juarez Tomas MS, Bru E, Wiese B, De Ruiz Holgado AA, Nader-Macias

ME. *Influence of pH, temperature and culture media on the growth and bacteriocin production by vaginal Lactobacillus salivarius* CRL 1328. J Appl Microbiol. 2002;93(4):714–24.

Kaur IP, Chopra K, Saini A. *Probiotics: potential pharmaceutical applications.* Eur J Pharm Sci. 2002 Feb;15(1):1–9. Review.

Kot E, Furmanov S, Berzkorovainy A. *Accumulation of iron in lactic acid bacteria and bifidobacteria.* Journal of Food Sciences. 1995;60(3):547–50.

Lykova EA, Vorob'ev AA, Bokovoi AG, Pobedinskaia IN, Gevondian VS, Gevondian NM, Mitrokhin SD, Minaev VI, Dzis NB, Makkaveeva LF, Kovalev IV, Murashova AO, Bondarenko VM. *Disruption of microbiocenosis of the large intestine and the immune and interferon status in children with bacterial complications of acute viral infections of the respiratory tract and their correction by high doses of bifidumbacterin forte.* Antibiot Khimioter. 2000;45(10):22–7. Russian.

Maia OB, Duarte R, Silva AM, Cara DC, Nicoli JR. *Evaluation of the components of a commercial probiotic in gnotobiotic mice experimentally challenged with Salmonella enterica subsp. enterica ser. Typhimurium.* Vet Microbiol. 2001 Mar 20;79(2):183–9.

Marteau P. *Probiotics in clinical conditions.* Clin Rev Allergy Immunol. 2002 Jun;22(3):255–73.

Marteau P, Boutron-Ruault MC. *Nutritional advantages of probiotics and prebiotics.* Br J Nutr. 2002 May;87 Suppl 2:S153–7.

Marteau P, Marteau P, Seksik P, Jian R. *Probiotics and intestinal health effects: A clinical perspective.* Br J Nutr. 2002 Sep;88 Suppl 1:S51–7.

Miller KS, Brudnak MA. *Expression cloning: PCR versus episomal vectors for rescue of transfected genes. In PCR in Neuroscience (Methods in Neuroscience, vol. 26)*, ed. G Sarkar. Academic Press, 1994.

Ochmanski W, Barabasz W. *Probiotics and their therapeutic properties.* Przegl Lek. 1999;56(3):211–5. Review. Polish.

Ouwehand AC, Salminen S, Isolauri E. *Probiotics: An overview of beneficial effects.* Antonie Van Leeuwenhoek. 2002 Aug;82(1-4):279–89.
Periti P, Tonelli F. Preclinical and clinical pharmacology of biotherapeutic

agents: Saccharomyces boulardii. J Chemother. 2001 Oct;13(5):473–93. Review.

Reid G. *Probiotic agents to protect the urogenital tract against infection.* Am J Clin Nutr. 2001 Feb;73(2 Suppl):437S–443S. Review.

Reid G. *Probiotics for urogenital health.* Nutr Clin Care. 2002 Jan–Feb;5(1):3–8. Review.

Sagen OB. *Treatment of functional disturbance in the intestine by administration of lactic acid bacteria.* Scand J Gastroenterol Suppl. 1989;109:59–68. Review.

Sipsas NV, Zonios DI, Kordossis T. *Safety of Lactobacillus strains used as probiotic agents.* Clin Infect Dis. 2002 May 1;34(9):1283–4; Discussion 1284–5.

Teitelbaum JE, Walker WA *Nutritional impact of pre- and probiotics as protective gastrointestinal organisms.* Annu Rev Nutr. 2002;22:107–38.

Van den Driessche M, Veereman-Wauters G. *Functional foods in pediatrics.* Acta Gastroenterol Belg. 2002 Jan–Mar;65(1):45–51. Review.

Varmanen P, Savijoki K, Avall S, Palva A, Tynkkynen S. *Related articles, links abstract X-prolyl dipeptidyl aminopeptidase gene (pepX) is part of the glnRA operon in Lactobacillus rhamnosus.* J Bacteriol. 2000 Jan;182(1):146–54.

Weber H, Vallett S, Neilson L, Chao Y, Grotke M, Brudnak MA, San Juan A, Pellegrini M. *Serum, insulin and phorbol esters stimulate rRNA and tRNA gene expression in both dividing and nondividing Drosophila cells.* Mol Cell Biochem. 1991 May 29–Jun 12;104(1–2):201–7.

Zegers ND, Kluter E, van Der Stap H, van Dura E, van Dalen P, Shaw M, Baillie L. *Expression of the protective antigen of Bacillus anthracis by Lactobacillus casei: Towards the development of an oral vaccine against anthrax.* J Appl Microbiol. 1999 Aug;87(2):309–14.

Zoppi G, Deganello A, Benoni G, Saccomani F. *Oral bacteriotherapy in clinical practice.* Eur J Pediatr. 1982 Sept.;139(1):18–21.

About the Author

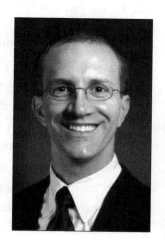

Mark A. Brudnak, Ph.D., N.D., is the author of over 40 peer-reviewed scientific and trade journal articles, written during his undergraduate study at the University of Southern California and continuing through his graduate study at the University of Tulsa. He is often quoted in the health food industry, cited in the peer-reviewed scientific literature, and sought out worldwide as a leading expert and speaker in the areas of probiotics, enzymes, and functional carbohydrates. He is the originator of the term *genomeceuticals*, which denotes the natural ingredients that beneficially affect gene expression. He is a member of many academic honor societies and has been the recipient of grants and scholarships throughout his career.

A board-certified naturopath, Brudnak has been involved with the natural products industry for over 15 years. He has worked with numerous companies and universities to develop novel products, many of which are available in local health food stores. He is the founder of Healthy Living Naturally, LLC, a natural health-consulting company that is also dedicated to the life extension of senior citizens through practicing the martial arts, such as TaeKwon-Do (TKD) and T'ai Chi Ch'uan. He has published a peer-reviewed journal article based on one of his studies on this topic. In addition to being on the faculty of the Association of Academies of Martial Arts (Grafton, WI), he has his own martial arts studio, Chosun TaeKwon-Do.

Brudnak has numerous personal interests. He is a poet as well as an accomplished pilot. He frequently offers free rides to disadvantaged youths, who would not ordinarily have the chance for such an outing. He also volunteers at a hospice, church, and senior citizens centers, and he donates time, energy, and money to finding cures for diseases such as autism and Down syndrome.

When asked why he wrote this book, Brudnak answered: "There is a need to bring the science of probiotics to the people, so that they can better their lives. Life is about balance, and I believe this book will help people balance themselves from the inside out. If one is not balanced on the inside, then it is impossible to be balanced on the outside. *The Probiotic Solution* shows both the importance of a balanced intestinal tract and how to balance the probiotics in it."

When asked about how to live life, he replied: " With courtesy, integrity, perseverance, self-control, and indomitable spirit. God, however you view Him, gives all of these gifts to us, if we look and believe."

Index

How to stay informed of the latest advances in diet and nutrition:

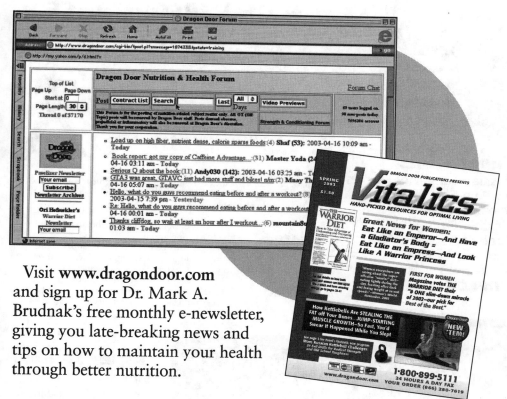

Visit **www.dragondoor.com** and sign up for Dr. Mark A. Brudnak's free monthly e-newsletter, giving you late-breaking news and tips on how to maintain your health through better nutrition.

Visit **www.dragondoor.com/cgi-bin/tpost.pl** and participate in Dragon Door's stimulating and informative Diet and Nutrition Forum. Post your diet questions or comments and get quick feedback from Dr. Mark A. Brudnak's and other leading nutrition experts.

Visit **www.dragondoor.com** and browse the Articles section and other pages for groundbreaking theories and products for improving your health and well being.

Call Dragon Door Publications at **1-800-899-5111** and request your FREE Vitalics catalog of fitness books, videos, supplements and equipment.

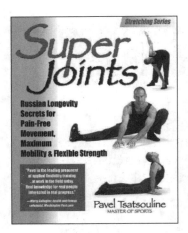

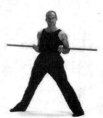

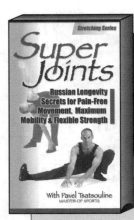

"The Do-It-Now, Fast-Start, Get-Up-and-Go, Jump-into-Action Bible for High Performance and Longer Life"

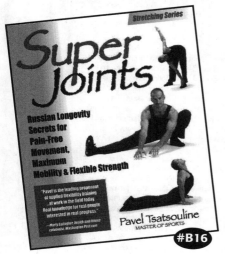

Super Joints
Russian Longevity Secrets for Pain-Free Movement, Maximum Mobility & Flexible Stength

With Pavel Tsatsouline
#B16   **$34.95**
8 1/2" x 11" Paperback
130 pages - Over 100 photos
and illustrations

You have a choice in life. You can sputter and stumble and creak your way along in a process of painful, slow decline—or you can take charge of your health and become a human dynamo.

And there is no better way to insure a long, pain-free life than performing the right daily combination of joint mobility and strength-flexibility exercises.

In *Super Joints*, Russian fitness expert Pavel Tsatsouline shows you exactly how to quickly achieve and maintain peak joint health—and then use it to improve every aspect of your physical performance.

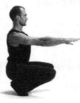

Only the foolish would deliberately ignore the life-saving and life-enhancing advice Pavel offers in *Super Joints*. Why would anyone willingly subject themselves

Discover:

- The twenty-eight most valuable drills for youthful joints and a stronger stretch
- How to save your joints and prevent or reduce arthritis
- The one-stop care-shop for your inner Tin Man— how to give your nervous system a tune up, your joints a lube-job and your energy a recharge
- What it takes to go from cruise control to full throttle: The One Thousand Moves Morning Recharge—Amosov's "bigger bang" calisthenics complex for achieving heaven-on earth in 25 minutes
- How to make your body feel better than you can remember— active flexibility fosporting

Manage Stress, Reduce Pain, Restore Energy, and Heal Yourself with the HIGHLY EFFECTIVE and PLEASURABLE METHODS of Chinese QIGONG

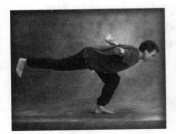

"John Du Cane has taken an ancient Chinese system, developed almost 2,000 years ago, and put together a practical and workable Qigong program for today's modern lifestyles. The Five Animals Frolics Qigong system is a series of exercises developed by ancient physicians that combines principles of Chinese medicine with shamanic healing systems. Its goal is to combine a wide range of movement, special breathing patterns, and visualization to awaken the internal power of self-healing. John Du Cane gives a strong demonstration of The Five Animals Frolics and clear instruction on each of these exercises that is beneficial to those beginning Qigong, as well as to seasoned practitioners."

—Rob Bracco, Editorial review for Amazon.com

"John Du Cane has created a good tape for learning some basic qigong practices. The instruction is clear and easily understood. The Bliss qigong movements are clearly explained in this tape, and are appropriate for beginners or experienced practitioners. Instructions are given in a logical fashion and at a pace that anyone can follow. His teaching style is gentle and the movements are not difficult to learn. His delivery is even and his manner inspires confidence. Along with teaching the movements, he includes information about qi and how it feels and functions in context of the exercises. There is not a lot of flash and glitter in the presentation, just straightforward instruction as if you were in the room with your teacher. This tape is easily among the best I have seen in the genre, and I would not hesitate to buy more of John Du Cane's works. I find the quality of his instruction to be in the same league as that of Ken Cohen and Chunyi Lin."

–Jon Norris, La Grande, OR

"One of the keys to success in life (as well as combat) is the ability to stay relaxed and focused. Many people struggle with this issue. I have seen people who are great practice athletes, but when competition time arrives, they become their worst nightmare. They get nervous and don't know how to channel this energy. The same is true in almost any endeavor. Knowing how to channel nervous

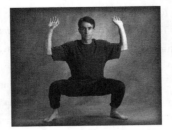

energy is a skill, and so is keeping your body relaxed. Even while you're reading this message, I'm sure most of you are using muscles that don't need to be doing anything. I'm also sure that most of you aren't breathing as deeply as you could be or should be. One thing that I have greatly benefited from over the years is the study of qigong or deep breathing exercises. I have done these exercises while holding still postures and I have done them while moving. It doesn't matter which way you do them, all that matters is that you are moving the energy in your body while staying relaxed and focused.

Recently I watched a NEW set of videotapes, produced by John Du Cane, on what is called "Five Animal Frolics Qigong." I tried to watch the tapes first to get an idea of what was on them, but it didn't take long for me to stop watching and start participating. Watching how gracefully John moved from one position to the next, and how relaxed he was, really got me thinking about how I needed to improve upon this skill as well. I especially liked the set of movements based upon the bear and the monkey. Really awesome. These movements generate POWER, that's for sure.

I highly recommend these tapes. Find out how to relax, reduce stress, increase power and energy, eliminate aches and pains, increase circulation and so on."

—Matt Furey, author of Combat Conditioning

"I felt completely CENTERED, FOCUSED, RELAXED and at PEACE, all accompanied by a VIBRANT SENSE OF ENERGY and WELL BEING."

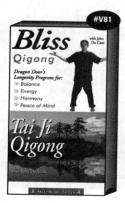
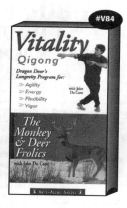
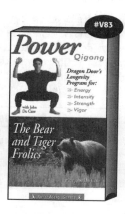
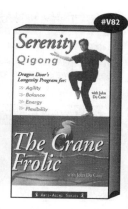

BLISS QIGONG
An instructional guide to Tai Ji Qigong

 # V81. 54 minutes. $29.95

Reveals the Yang Family's personal qigong program, with additional tips on energy accumulation and balancing. The simple movements gently harmonize the qi, promote blood circulation, cultivate vitality, regulate the breath and reduce stress.

Discover:
- How to use attention to effectively feel and direct qi
- How to activate all your major energy centers
- How to turn on healing power in your hands
- How to clear all the major meridians in your body
- How to develop your sensing ability
- How to get real results with you standing qigong practice
- How to incorporate special internal sounds to deepen your meditation

VITALITY QIGONG
An instructional guide to The Monkey and Deer Frolics

 # V84. 43 minutes. $29.95

The Monkey develops suppleness, agility, and quick wit, training you to remain alert and calm, even as you are outwardly spirited and mobile. The Deer gives a long stretch to the legs and spine, creating open, expansive movement with very flexible sinews and bones. The Deer embodies grace and relaxation, while regulating the endocrine system.

Discover:
- How to flood your system with warming qi
- How to quickly improve your muscle tone
- How to develop strong, mobile joints

POWER QIGONG
An instructional guide to The Bear and Tiger Frolics

 # V83. 48 minutes. $29.95

The Bear is a great winter exercise. Slow, ponderous, but very strong, it warms the body, strengthens the spleen, and builds vitality. The Bear's twisting waist movements massage and invigorate the kidneys. The Bear is an excellent preventive against osteoporosis, as it is known to fortify the bones. The dynamic Tiger builds great power, strengthening your waist, sinews, and kidneys and developing you internally.

Discover:
- How to develop power and strength
- How to generate coiling energy
- How to develop a strong root

SERENITY QIGONG
An instructional guide to The Crane Frolic

 # V82. 41 minutes. $29.95

Practice an invigorating mix of dynamic and tranquil postures for self-healing and athletic grace. The Crane develops balance, lightness, and agility, releases the spine, and relaxes your whole body.

Discover:
- How to absorb qi from the universe for self-healing
- How to extend your qi beyond your own body
- How to develop balanced leg strength
- How to heal your lungs

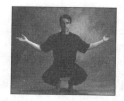

1. Improve your metabolism, digestion, and elimination—for weight control, more youthful appearance, and higher, longer-lasting energy.

2. Stimulate the lymph system—for a stronger immune system. Be less susceptible to the flu or colds and recover faster if you do get sick.

3. Improve your circulation—alleviating conditions such as arthritis and chronic fatigue.

4. Build stronger, more durable bones.

5. Give your internal organs an "inner massage"—retarding the aging process by restoring your organs to peak efficiency.

6. Increase oxygen in the tissues—reducing tensions, blocks and stagnant energy.

7. Lubricate the joints—for pain free movement and greater flexibility.

8. Soothe the nervous system—for feelings of contentment and serenity.

ORDERING INFORMATION

Customer Service Questions? Please call us between 9:00am– 11:00pm EST Monday to Friday at 1-800-899-5111. Local and foreign customers call 513-346-4160 for orders and customer service

100% One-Year Risk-Free Guarantee. If you are not completely satisfied with any product–for any reason, no matter how long after you received it–we'll be happy to give you a prompt exchange, credit, or refund, as you wish. Simply return your purchase to us, and please let us know why you were dissatisfied–it will help us to provide better products and services in the future. *Shipping and handling fees are non-refundable.*

Telephone Orders For faster service you may place your orders by calling Toll Free 24 hours a day, 7 days a week, 365 days per year. When you call, please have your credit card ready.

1·800·899·5111
24 HOURS A DAY
FAX YOUR ORDER (866) 280-7619

Complete and mail with full payment to: Dragon Door Publications, P.O. Box 1097, West Chester, OH 45071

Please print clearly

Sold To: A

Name_____

Street_____

City_____

State _____ Zip _____

Day phone*_____
* Important for clarifying questions on orders

Please print clearly

SHIP TO: *(Street address for delivery)*   B

Name_____

Street_____

City_____

State _____ Zip _____

Email_____

Warning to foreign customers:
The Customs in your country may or may not tax or otherwise charge you an additional fee for goods you receive. Dragon Door Publications is charging you only for U.S. handling and international shipping. Dragon Door Publications is in no way responsible for any additional fees levied by Customs, the carrier or any other entity.

Warning!
This may be the last issue of the catalog you receive.

If we rented your name, or you haven't ordered in the last two years you may not hear from us again. If you wish to stay informed about products and services that can make a difference to your health and well-being, please indicate below.

Name_____

Address_____

City_____ State_____

Zip_____

Item #	Qty.	Item Description	Item Price	A or B	Total

HANDLING AND SHIPPING CHARGES • NO COD'S

Total Amount of Order Add:

$00.00 to $24.99	add $5.00	$100.00 to $129.99	add $12.00
$25.00 to $39.99	add $6.00	$130.00 to $169.99	add $14.00
$40.00 to $59.99	add $7.00	$170.00 to $199.99	add $16.00
$60.00 to $99.99	add $10.00	$200.00 to $299.99	add $18.00
		$300.00 and up	add $20.00

Canada & Mexico add $8.00. All other countries triple U.S. charges.

Total of Goods	
Shipping Charges	
Rush Charges	
Kettlebell Shipping Charges	
OH residents add 6% sales tax	
MN residents add 6.5% sales tax	
Total Enclosed	

Do You Have A Friend Who'd Like To Receive This Catalog?

We would be happy to send your friend a free copy. Make sure to print and complete in full:

Name_____

Address_____

City_____ State_____

Zip_____

Method of Payment ☐ Check ☐ M.O. ☐ Mastercard ☐ Visa ☐ Discover ☐ Amex

Account No. *(Please indicate all the numbers on your credit card)*   EXPIRATION DATE

☐☐☐☐ ☐☐☐☐ ☐☐☐☐ ☐☐☐☐   ☐☐/☐☐

Day Phone ( )_____

SIGNATURE_____ DATE _____

NOTE: We ship best method available for your delivery address. Foreign orders are sent by air. Credit card or International M.O. only. For rush processing of your order, add an additional $10.00 per address. Available on money order & charge card orders only.

Errors and omissions excepted. Prices subject to change without notice.

DDP 04/03

ORDERING INFORMATION

Customer Service Questions? Please call us between 9:00am– 11:00pm EST Monday to Friday at 1-800-899-5111. Local and foreign customers call 513-346-4160 for orders and customer service

Telephone Orders For faster service you may place your orders by calling Toll Free 24 hours a day, 7 days a week, 365 days per year. When you call, please have your credit card ready.

100% One-Year Risk-Free Guarantee. If you are not completely satisfied with any product–for any reason, no matter how long after you received it–we'll be happy to give you a prompt exchange, credit, or refund, as you wish. Simply return your purchase to us, and please let us know why you were dissatisfied–it will help us to provide better products and services in the future. *Shipping and handling fees are non-refundable.*

1·800·899·5111
24 HOURS A DAY
FAX YOUR ORDER (866) 280-7619

Complete and mail with full payment to: Dragon Door Publications, P.O. Box 1097, West Chester, OH 45071

Please print clearly

Sold To: A

Name_____

Street_____

City_____

State_____ Zip_____

Day phone*_____

* Important for clarifying questions on orders

Please print clearly

SHIP TO: *(Street address for delivery)*   B

Name_____

Street_____

City_____

State_____ Zip_____

Email_____

Warning to foreign customers:

The Customs in your country may or may not tax or otherwise charge you an additional fee for goods you receive. Dragon Door Publications is charging you only for U.S. handling and international shipping. Dragon Door Publications is in no way responsible for any additional fees levied by Customs, the carrier or any other entity.

Item #	Qty.	Item Description	Item Price	A or B	Total

Warning!
This may be the last issue of the catalog you receive.

If we rented your name, or you haven't ordered in the last two years you may not hear from us again. If you wish to stay informed about products and services that can make a difference to your health and well-being, please indicate below.

Name..

Address..

City........................ State..............

Zip..

HANDLING AND SHIPPING CHARGES • NO COD'S

Total Amount of Order Add:

$00.00 to $24.99 add $5.00	$100.00 to $129.99 add $12.00
$25.00 to $39.99 add $6.00	$130.00 to $169.99 add $14.00
$40.00 to $59.99 add $7.00	$170.00 to $199.99 add $16.00
$60.00 to $99.99 add $10.00	$200.00 to $299.99 add $18.00
	$300.00 and up add $20.00

Canada & Mexico add $8.00. All other countries triple U.S. charges.

Total of Goods	
Shipping Charges	
Rush Charges	
Kettlebell Shipping Charges	
OH residents add 6% sales tax	
MN residents add 6.5% sales tax	
Total Enclosed	

METHOD OF PAYMENT ❑ CHECK ❑ M.O. ❑ MASTERCARD ❑ VISA ❑ DISCOVER ❑ AMEX

Account No. *(Please indicate all the numbers on your credit card)*   EXPIRATION DATE

❑❑❑❑ ❑❑❑❑ ❑❑❑❑ ❑❑❑❑   ❑❑/❑❑

Day Phone (   )_____

SIGNATURE_____ DATE_____

NOTE: We ship best method available for your delivery address. Foreign orders are sent by air. Credit card or International M.O. only. For rush processing of your order, add an additional $10.00 per address. Available on money order & charge card orders only.

Errors and omissions excepted. Prices subject to change without notice.

Do You Have A Friend Who'd Like To Receive This Catalog?

We would be happy to send your friend a free copy. Make sure to print and complete in full:

Name..

Address..

City........................ State..............

Zip....................................   DDP 04/03